Alcohol-induced liver disease is the most common cause of end-stage liver failure in the developed world, and liver transplantation has become an increasingly common form of treatment in such patients. This poses especially difficult dilemmas for health care workers in liver transplant programs.

This text provides a scientific and scholarly review of the medical, surgical and psychosocial aspects of evaluation, surgery and post-transplant care in this group. A unique synthesis of the three distinct clinical disciplines involved in optimal management of these patients, it draws on the extensive experience gained in recent years at the University of Michigan Medical Center.

Practical advice is given on the clinical and social problems encountered, and the text is enlivened by the use of case vignettes drawn from the authors' own experience. The book concludes with a stimulating discussion of the ethical issues surrounding the controversial topic of liver transplantation in alcoholics. Essential reading for all involved in organ transplantation, it will provide valuable insights to all physicians, surgeons, psychiatrists and related health care professionals involved in the care of alcoholic patients.

LIVER TRANSPLANTATION & THE ALCOHOLIC PATIENT: MEDICAL, SURGICAL AND PSYCHOSOCIAL ISSUES

LIVER TRANSPLANTATION & THE ALCOHOLIC PATIENT: MEDICAL, SURGICAL AND PSYCHOSOCIAL ISSUES

Michael R. Lucey

Associate Professor of Internal Medicine, Division of Gastroenterology, Department of Internal Medicine, Medical Director, Liver Transplant Program, University of Michigan, Ann Arbor, USA

Robert M. Merion

Chief Division of Transplantation, Associate Professor of Surgery, University of Michigan, Medical School, Ann Arbor, USA

Thomas P. Beresford

Professor of Psychiatry, University of Colorado School of Medicine, the Veterans Affairs Alcohol Research Center and the University of Colorado Alcohol Research Center, Denver, USA

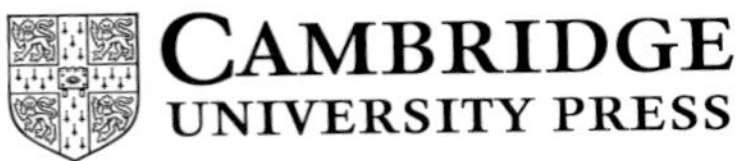
CAMBRIDGE UNIVERSITY PRESS

Published by the Press Syndicate of the University of Cambridge
The Pitt Building, Trumpington Street, Cambridge CB2 1RP
40 West 20th Street, New York, NY 10011-4211, USA
10 Stamford Road, Oakleigh, Melbourne 3166, Australia

First published 1994

Printed in Great Britain at the University Press, Cambridge

A catalogue record for this book is available from the British Library

Library of Congress cataloguing in publication data

Liver transplantation & the alcoholic patient : medical, surgical and psychosocial issues / Michael R. Lucey, Robert M. Merion, Thomas P. Beresford.
p. cm.
Includes index.
ISBN (invalid) 0-521-43332-0 (hardback)
1. Liver – Transplantation. 2. Alcoholic liver diseases – Surgery.
3. Liver – Transplantation – Moral and ethical aspects. 4. Ethics, Medical. I. Lucey, Michael R. II. Merion, Robert M.
III. Beresford, Thomas P.
[DNLM: 1. Liver Transplantation. 2. Liver Diseases, Alcoholic – surgery.
3. Liver Diseases, Alcoholic – psychology. WI 725 L784 1994]
RD546.L563 1994
617.5'56 – dc20 93-24229 CIP

ISBN 0 521 43332 0 hardback

TAG

CONTENTS

CONTRIBUTORS

Martin Benjamin, PhD
Department of Philosophy
Michigan State University
503 South Kedzie Hall
East Lansing,
Michigan 48824-1032
USA

Thomas P. Beresford, MD
Department of Psychiatry
University of Colorado School of Medicine
Psychiatry Service (116A)
Veteran's Administration Medical Center
1055 Clermont Street
Denver,
Colorado 80220-3977
USA

Michael R. Lucey, MD, FRCPI
Department of Internal Medicine
University of Michigan Medical Center
3912 Taubman Center, Box 0362
Ann Arbor,
Michigan 48109-0362
USA

Robert M. Merion, MD
Department of Surgery
University of Michigan Medical Center
2926F Taubman Center
Ann Arbor,
Michigan 48109-0331
USA

Jeremiah G. Turcotte, MD
Department of Surgery
University of Michigan Medical Center
2924F Taubman Center
Ann Arbor,
Michigan 48109-0331
USA

PREFACE

This monograph has two broad aims: first to offer a scholarly review of all aspects of liver transplantation in persons affected by alcoholism, and second to provide a practical guide for health care professionals involved in the selection of alcoholics for liver transplantation and their management after transplantation. In this, we have drawn on the experience we have gained as members of the University of Michigan liver transplant program. We did not confine ourselves to our own data. We have reviewed the psychiatric and medical aspects of alcoholism, mechanisms of alcohol-induced liver injury, management of end-stage liver disease and the early and late postoperative management of liver transplantation recipients wherever these topics fall within the two broad aims described above. However, this text is not an exhaustive review of alcoholism, alcoholic liver disease or liver transplantation in general. Finally, the monograph contains a review of the ethics of liver transplantation for alcoholic liver disease, written by two colleagues who have taken a special interest in this important topic.

We are grateful for the support given to this project by three alcohol research centers located in the Universities of Michigan and Colorado and at the Veteran's Affairs Medical Center, Denver, Colorado. This work could not have been completed without the assistance of the National Institute on Alcohol Abuse and Alcoholism through its extramural grants P50-AA-07378 and RO1-AA-07236 that supported Dr Beresford's researches. Furthermore, we acknowledge our many colleagues in the University of Michigan Liver Transplant Program and all the patients we have cared for in the Program. They have contributed immeasurably to the development of the ideas presented in this book. The imperfections in the material presented, however, are the sole responsibility of the authors.

We would like to thank Evonne LaVigne, Julie Knight and JoAnn Suriskey for valuable secretarial assistance. We are grateful to the staff of Cambridge University Press for their help and cooperation. Finally, we would like to acknowledge the encouragement and forbearance of our wives and families during the preparation of this monograph.

M. R. Lucey
R. M. Merion
T. P. Beresford

CHAPTER ONE

AN OVERVIEW

MICHAEL R. LUCEY

Historical background

Alcohol-induced liver disease is the most common cause of end-stage liver failure in the developed world (Zakim *et al.*, 1990). Nonetheless, until recently, alcoholic liver disease was an unusual preoperative diagnosis among patients undergoing liver transplantation in the USA (Scharschmidt, 1984) and Europe (Bismuth *et al.*, 1987). This was in part due to early reports of a poor outcome when alcoholics received liver transplants (Scharschmidt, 1984). The latter data were seriously flawed, however, by being based on the outcome of liver transplantation in 25 patients in whom neither the diagnosis of alcoholism and alcoholic liver disease nor the reasons for their selection were adequately defined.

A second reason for the rarity of recognized alcoholics among patients receiving liver transplants in the decade from 1975 to 1985 was the view that alcoholics with end-stage liver disease should undergo a more stringent process of selection than non-alcoholics. This opinion continues to have its advocates today (Moss and Siegler, 1991) and will be discussed in detail in Chapter 7. It was also suggested that alcoholics were inherently unsuitable for liver transplantation because they were at such a high risk to continue alcohol abuse after transplantation thereby leading to non-compliance with post-transplant management (Schenker, 1983). The authors of the influential National Institutes of Health Consensus Conference on liver transplantation, while acknowledging that 'patients (with alcoholic liver disease) who are judged likely to abstain from alcohol and have established clinical indicators of fatal outcomes may be candidates for transplantation', at the same time asserted that 'only a small proportion of alcoholic patients with liver disease would be expected to meet the rigorous criteria' (Anonymous, 1984). Subsequent studies, which will be discussed in detail in this volume, have not confirmed either the predicted dismal outcome of liver transplantation in alcoholics or that few alcoholics are selected for transplantation when rigorous selection criteria are applied.

Success of liver transplantation for alcoholic liver disease

In 1988, Starzl *et al.* reported an estimated 1 year survival of 73.2% in 41 alcoholic patients undergoing liver transplantation in Pittsburgh between 1980 and 1987 (Starzl *et al.*, 1988). We have recently reported an actuarial survival after liver transplantation among 45 patients with carefully defined alcoholic liver disease of 78% and 73% at 12 and 24 months, respectively (Lucey *et al.*, 1992). In Chapter 5, Merion expands these data to include 90 alcoholics transplanted at the University of Michigan. Once again, the outcome does not differ from that in non-alcoholic adult patients who received liver transplants during the same period of time. The medical and psychiatric selection process which we have used will be described in detail in subsequent chapters. It is clear that among carefully selected alcoholics with end-stage liver disease, liver transplantation is at least as efficacious as in non-alcoholic patients with severe non-alcoholic liver disease.

Liver transplantation has never been subjected to a controlled clinical trial. The ethical issues arising from clinical trials of potentially life saving therapies are well discussed by Hellman and Hellman, and Passamami (Hellman and Hellman, 1991; Passamami, 1991). An essential requirement for an ethical clinical trial is equipoise – a state of uncertainty on the part of the investigator, or within the scientific community, about the comparative therapeutic merits of each arm of the trial (Freedman, 1987). This is not possible with liver transplantation owing to the conviction within the transplantation community that liver transplantation gives substantially better results than medical management for many patients with advanced end stage liver disease. These difficulties have prevented a controlled clinical trial in the use of liver transplantation to manage fulminant hepatic failure for example (Chapman *et al.*, 1990).

Despite the absence of randomized placebo-controlled trial data, this book will argue from the proposition that liver transplantation is an efficacious remedy for, at least, some patients with alcoholic liver disease.

Our conviction that liver transplantation is an efficacious treatment of end-stage liver disease in alcoholics is supported by the survival advantage of alcoholics selected for liver transplantation compared with alcoholic cirrhotics who were declined transplantation on psychiatric grounds (Lucey *et al.*, 1992) (Figure 4.6). The two cohorts in this study had similar Child–Pugh classes suggesting that they had a similar degree of liver dysfunction. Thus the best data available, albeit not derived from a controlled trial, suggest that transplantation is a valuable therapy in patients with decompensated alcoholic liver disease.

Selection for liver transplantation

Liver transplantation is dependent upon a gift. We, the facilitators of a liver transplant program, have responsibilities to both the potential recipient and the gift giver. Our primary responsibility is to provide the best care for our patients. Our secondary responsibility is to allocate the donated liver with prudence. The philosophic foundation of our transplantation program rests on the view that selection for liver transplantation should be made with regard to medical necessity and the potential for a successful outcome and should be independent of diagnosis. This is particularly so in the case of alcoholic liver disease (Lucey and Beresford, 1992).

In subsequent chapters we describe in detail the process of selection that we have devised. It involves answering three questions. (1) Does the patient have significant liver disease for which liver transplantation is the best treatment? (2) Are there any other factors in the patients health which would prevent a successful outcome? Confounding factors could be medical, such as disseminated cancer or heart failure; or surgical, such as extensive clot in the portal venous system. Portal vein occlusion, however, is rarely an absolute contraindication of transplantation. A poor prognosis for maintaining abstinence from alcohol after liver transplantation is considered to be a contraindication to transplantation because it is likely to lead to poor compliance with the post-transplant immunosuppressive regimen. In Chapter 4, Beresford describes in detail how we have attempted to predict future psychiatric morbidity in alcoholic patients undergoing evaluation for liver transplantation. In the course of this description, he draws on the experience gained at the University of Michigan to include actual case vignettes to illustrate practical clinical points.

(3) Does the patient wish to undergo liver transplantation if it is the consensus of the evaluation committee that a transplant is appropriate? We have developed a well-organized program of education to inform the patient and their family of the risks and benefits of liver transplantation to assist them in making these decisions.

Long-term outcome and management of alcoholics with liver transplants

As mentioned above, recent experience at the University of Michigan and other centers has not confirmed the earlier predictions that alcoholic persons would have a lower survival after liver transplantation than non-alcoholic recipients (Kumar *et al.*, 1992; Lucey *et al.*, 1990). Current research is looking beyond survival to the quality of life after transplantation. Data from the University of Michigan suggest that short-term psychiatric morbidity is similar in alcoholics and non-alcoholics (Beresford *et al.* 1992). We review in detail mortality and morbidity in alcoholics who receive liver transplantation. Special attention is given to the incidence and management of recidivism.

References

Anonymous. (1984). National Institutes of Health Consensus Development Conference Statement: Liver transplantation. *Hepatology*, **4**, 1075–105.

Beresford, T.P., Wilson, D., Blow, F.C., Hill, E., Merion, R.M., and Lucey, M.R. (1992). Short-term psychological health in alcoholic and non-alcoholic liver transplant recipients. *Alcoholism, Clinical and Experimental Research*, **16**, 996–1000.

Bismuth, H., Castaing, D., Ericzon, B.G., Otte, J.B., Rolles, K., Ringe, B. and Sloof, M. (1987). Hepatic Transplantation in Europe. First report of the European liver transplant registry. *Lancet*, **ii**, 674–6.

Chapman, R.W., Forman, D., Peto, R., and Smallwood, R. (1990). Liver transplantation for acute hepatic failure? *Lancet*, **335**, 32–5.

Freedman, B. (1987). Equipoise and the ethics of clinical research. *New England Journal of Medicine*, **317**, 141–5.

Hellman, S. and Hellman, D. (1991). Of mice but not men: Problems of the randomized clinical trial. *New England Journal of Medicine*, **324**, 1585–9.

Kumar, S., Staubet, R.E., Gavaler, J.S., Basista, M.H., Dindzans, V.J., Schade, R.R., Rabinovitz, M., Tarter, R.E., Gordon, R., Starzl, T.E. and VanThiel, D.H. (1990). Orthotopic liver transplantation for alcoholic liver disease. *Hepatology*, **11**, 159–64.

Lucey, M.R. and Beresford, T.P. (1992). Alcoholic liver disease: to transplant or not to transplant? *Alcohol & Alcoholism*, **27**, 103–8.

Lucey, M.R., Merion, R.M., Henley, K.S., Campbell, D.A., Turcotte, J.G., Nostrant,

T.T., Blow, F.C. and Beresford, T.P. (1992). Selection for and outcome of liver transplantation in alcoholic liver disease. *Gastroenterology*, **102**, 1736–41.

Moss, A.H. and Siegler, M. (1991). Should alcoholics compete equally for liver transplantation? *Journal of the American Medical Association*, **265**, 1295–8.

Passamani, E. (1991). Clinical trials – are they ethical? *New England Journal of Medicine*, **324**, 1589–92.

Scharschmidt, B.F. (1984). Human liver transplantation: analysis of data on 540 patients from 4 centers. *Hepatology*, **4**, 95S–111S.

Schenker, S. (1984). Medical treatment versus transplantation in liver disorders. *Hepatology*, **4**, 102S–106S.

Starzl, T.E., VanThiel, D., Tzakis, A.G., Iwatsuki, S., Todo, S., Marsh, J.W., Koneru, B., Staschak, S., Stieber, A. and Gordon, R.D. (1988). Orthotopic liver transplantation for alcoholic cirrhosis. *Journal of the American Medical Association*, **260**, 2542–4.

Zakim, D., Boyer, T.D. and Montgomery, C. (1990). Alcoholic liver disease. In *Hepatology*. A Textbook of Liver Disease; 2nd edn, Vol. 2, eds. D. Zakim and T.D. Boyer, pp. 821–68. Philadelphia: W.B. Saunders.

CHAPTER TWO

OVERT AND COVERT ALCOHOLISM

THOMAS P. BERESFORD

Introduction

Alcoholism afflicts some 7–10% of Americans at some time in their lives. (Vaillant, 1983). About 15% of persons suffering from alcoholism will develop alcoholic cirrhosis (Zakim *et al.*, 1989), the most frequent cause of liver failure in the USA today (Grant *et al.*, 1991). In real numbers, about one to two million Americans suffer from alcoholic cirrhosis at any one time. Approximately 3000 human livers are transplanted in the USA each year and to provide liver grafts for alcoholic cirrhotics would overwhelm current resources. The cost of the procedure is high and the availability of organs suitable for transplantation is low, thus requiring the judicious conservation of this life saving resource.

Transplant teams must face the difficult responsibility of selecting patients for liver transplant because of these constraints. A part of this responsibility is the need to apply our clinical knowledge of alcoholism with the greatest possible precision to the problem of patient selection. The difficulty lies in the often murky field of alcohol studies itself, in which differing views of the same phenomenon compete and in which clinicians, acting in good faith, may arrive at opposing conclusions. This chapter, and the subsequent chapters on evaluation and follow-up care of alcoholics undergoing liver transplantation, will emphasize the practical over the theoretical, the operational approaches over the disciplinary nuances, and general consensus over parochial points of view. In addition to our own experience, the experience of others reported here (e.g. Surman, 1989) will, hopefully, shed light on this difficult subject.

What does 'alcoholism' mean?

Alcoholism is generally taken to refer to a condition in which someone regularly drinks more ethyl alcohol than is good for them. This may mean chronic drunkenness, harm to one's self or to someone else because of drinking, or the downhill slide from social and personal well-being to loneliness, illness and death that often goes hand-in-hand with chronic, heavy drinking. This general view of alcoholism may contain much truth but in a practical sense it does not offer sufficient precision to be applied clinically. In recent years, therefore, other definitions of alcoholism and its various forms have been proposed. This has allowed operational definitions that can be used in empirical research to test the validity and reliability of such concepts. In this discussion we will consider two operational definitions of 'alcoholism': alcohol dependence and alcohol abuse. A third definition or clinical form will also be considered briefly: alcoholism in the setting of poly-drug dependence.

Early researchers began to distinguish various subgroups of what appeared to be different types of alcoholics. These subgroups were distinguishable by the presence or absence of four key features, notably: (1) tolerance to alcohol, (2) withdrawal symptoms on ceasing alcohol use, (3) indications of an inability to control drinking once drinking began, and (4) untoward social or physical consequences resulting from alcohol use. As an example, Table 2.1 presents an operationalized version of the criteria for alcohol dependence adapted from standard criteria for substance dependence (DSM-III-R, 1987).

Dependence on alcohol has generally been construed in two ways. The first is physical dependence, which denotes the presence of tolerance and withdrawal symptoms. (Table 2.1C). For some, physical dependence is a necessary but not sufficient condition for the diagnosis of alcohol dependence whereas for others

Table 2.1. *DSM-III-R diagnostic criteria*

Construed as Domains Specific To Alcohol Dependence
A. *Impaired control*
(1) Alcohol often taken in larger amounts or over a longer period than the person intends
(2) Persistent desire or one or more unsuccessful efforts to cut down or control alcohol use
(3) A great deal of time spent in activities necessary to get alcohol, take alcohol, or recover from its effects
B. *Social/physical sequelae*
(4) Frequent intoxication or withdrawal symptoms when expected to fulfill major role obligations at work, school, or home (e.g., does not go to work because hung over, goes to school or work with alcohol on board, intoxicated while taking care of his or her children), or when substance use is physically hazardous (e.g. drives when intoxicated)
(5) Important social, occupational or recreational activities given up or reduced because of alcohol use
(6) Continued alcohol use despite knowledge of having a persistent or recurrent social, psychological or physical problem that is caused or exacerbated by the use of alcohol (e.g. keeps using alcohol despite family arguments about it, alcohol-induced depression or having an ulcer made worse by drinking)
C. *Physical dependence*
(7) Marked tolerance: need for markedly increased amounts of alcohol (i.e. at least a 50% increase) in order to achieve intoxication or desired effect or markedly diminished effect with continued use of the same amount
(8) Characteristic alcohol withdrawal symptoms
(9) Alcohol often taken to relieve or avoid withdrawal symptoms

it is one of a series of symptom categories that, when summed, indicate this diagnosis.

The second type of dependence is psychological dependence, which for many persons is an insatiable need to imbibe alcohol whether because of a subjective effect of the alcohol or because of a pattern of habitual use; because of this, psychological dependence has often included the idea of craving for alcohol. For those who systematically study alcoholic behavior, craving appears in one of two forms. The first is craving for a drink when a drinking episode has already begun, and the second is craving for a drink between drinking episodes. The former is more common by far and has been codified as the 'loss-of-control' or 'impaired-control' phenomenon (Table 2.1A). The latter is regarded as a less predictable occurrence and is currently spoken of in the literature that discusses alcoholic relapse or relapse prevention. For the purposes of diagnosis, the loss-of-control phenomenon has become an important facet of diagnosis whereas some regard relapse behavior more as part of the natural course of this condition (Vaillant, 1983).

Recent codification schemes have provided more generally useful means of diagnosing alcohol dependence. The standard instrument at present in the USA is the Diagnostic and Statistical Manual (DSM-III-R, 1987) definition of substance dependency. As exemplified in Table 2.1, the DSM-III-R requires the clinician to assess each of nine symptom categories and then to decide whether the patient satisfied any three of those symptom categories. An earlier version (DSM-III, 1980), required some evidence of physical dependence, either tolerance or withdrawal, together with evidence of either loss of control of drinking or social difficulties after alcohol use.* The current approach dispenses with this prerequisite and a person may be diagnosed as alcohol dependent solely on the basis of any three symptoms which may be derived from the same general category. The reader will note that the first three symptom categories relate to the impaired-control or loss-of-control phenomenon, that the second triad assesses social, physical or personal decline, and that the final three symptom categories chart aspects of physical dependence.

While the DSM-III-R criteria are the standard in the USA, the ICD-10 criteria serve the same role in many European countries. Viewed from a great distance, both standards require evidence of physical dependence, impaired control and social/physical decline, i.e. each of the three symptom domains are represented but viewed close up, the specific criteria by which the symptom domains are assessed vary both in emphasis and in kind (Table 2.2). It is theoretically possible either for a patient diagnosed as alcoholic on one side of the Atlantic to lose that label after a transoceanic voyage or to gain the diagnosis in the same way. In this field, as perhaps in few others, reliance on the judgment of seasoned clinicians and, where possible, on more than one or two clinical observations, is very important.

In Table 2.3, we list our experience with 1139 patients admitted randomly to general medical and surgical wards in a university hospital from whom we systematically gathered clinical histories of alcohol use. We construed these histories into various diagnostic schema, those mentioned above as well as others

* In one version of a proposed update of this schema (DSM-IV), physical dependence will once again be required as necessary for the diagnosis of alcohol dependence, along with some combination of other symptom domains. See Table 2.3.

Table 2.2. *Comparison of two alcohol dependence criteria*

DSM-III-R criteria	ICD-10 criteria
1. Drinking > intent	2. Awareness of impaired control
2. Unable to cut down/stop use	2. Awareness of impaired control
3. Much time used to get/use/recover	No counterpart
4. Use despite obligations or hazards	No counterpart
5. Activities given up because of drinking	7. Neglect of alternative pleasures
6. Continued use despite problems	8. Persistent use despite harm
7. Marked tolerance	5. Evidence of tolerance
8. Characteristic withdrawal symptoms	4. Physiological withdrawal state
9. Alcohol use to treat withdrawal	3. Alcohol effective for withdrawal
No counterpart	1. Desire/compulsion to drink
No counterpart	6. Narrowing drinking pattern
No counterpart	9. Relapse leads to rapid return of symptoms

Source: adapted from Atkinson (1990).

proffered by Cahalan and by Vaillant. The Cahalan scale (Cahalan, 1970) was derived from a large national telephone survey that contained a preponderance of questions assessing social problems due to alcohol. Vaillant's Problem Drinking Scale (Vaillant, 1983) was used longitudinally to describe a clinical sample of alcoholics and included measures of physical dependence and loss of control in addition to social difficulties. There is some variation from one diagnostic scheme to the next when considering this same sample. Each of the 'DSM' constructions approximate the rate found in the others, but the rates vary by as much as 10–15%. While this may be of small significance in large community surveys of persons who are not suffering the immediate catastrophic consequences of their alcoholism, variations in diagnostic validity of this size may be more disturbing for the clinicians who are engaged in life or death decision making.

The problem of diagnosis worsens when one considers the leeway *within* the standard USA definition itself. Some symptom categories have only one alternative answer, as for example category number 9, in which a person either does or does not engage in morning drinking to get rid of a hangover. Other categories can have many possible answers, such as category number 4, which assesses the different social problems arising from alcohol use. Figure 2.1, taken from our work (Beresford *et al.*, 1991), depicts prevalence frequencies of DSM-III-R alcohol dependence in the same hospital sample based on four different approaches to weighting the three diagnostic domains (Table 2.1 A–C) and the nine diagnostic categories (Table 2.1, 1-9). In the first approach we

Table 2.3. *Comparisons of prevalences of alcohol dependence or abuse criteria among a general hospital patient sample*

Dependence or abuse criteria	Prevalence (%)
DSM-III-R dependence	34
DSM-III	
Abuse	14
Dependence	25
DSM-IV dependence, proposed	30
Cahalan scale	
Two or more problems	30
Four or more problems	13
Problem drinking scale	
Two or more problems	40
Four or more problems	19

n =1139 medical/surgical inpatients.

counted those subjects who presented at least one positive response for any three of the nine symptom criteria (liberal). In this scheme, over one-third of our patients merited a diagnosis of alcohol dependence. In the next approach (L-domains) we required at least one positive response in each of the three symptom domains: loss of control, social or physical decline and physical dependence. The prevalence rate fell to 27%. We next required any three positive of the nine diagnostic criteria but added the constraint of at least two positive phenomenon in those categories in which more than one choice was possible (Strict), the prevalence rate fell again to 23%. Finally, by requiring evidence in all three symptom domains together with more than one positive response in any symptom category with multiple possible responses (S-domains), the prevalence rate fell to 16% or approximately half of the prevalence when we used the DSM-III-R criteria as written.

There is a lesson in this exercise: each clinician or team of clinicians must acquire sufficient experience with this diagnosis, in the form that they find most clinically defensible, and use that diagnostic approach consistently in evaluating potential transplant patients. We have preferred the more conservative scheme of requiring evidence of tolerance and withdrawal, of the loss-of-control phenomenon, and of social or physical decline, before assigning a diagnosis of alcohol dependence. The reason derives from a decision to err on the side of a conservative diagnosis rather than to risk loss of life because of a misdiagnosis.

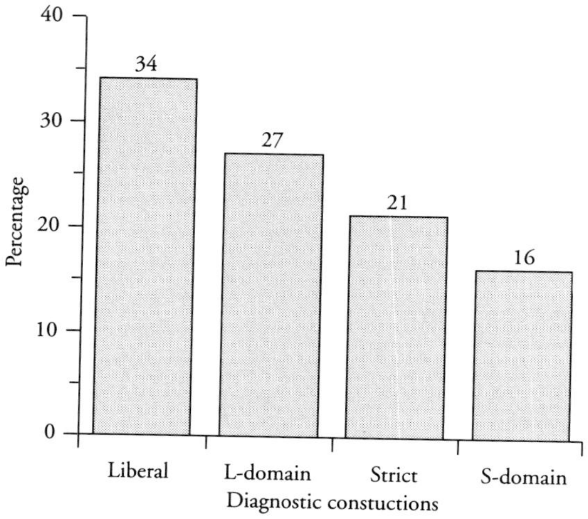

Figure 2.1. Applications of DSM-III-R criteria resulting in prevalences of alcoholic dependence in 1146 random medical/surgical inpatients.

Table 2.4 lists our experience with this diagnostic approach. In contrast to alcohol *dependence* we have taken alcohol *abuse* to mean a very specific syndrome (DSM-III, 1980) in which a patient presents with a clear history of tolerance to alcohol in the absence of any other symptoms of dependence. In our experience, alcohol abuse has presented in this way, as corroborated by a family member, in a little more than 10% of patients. Surprisingly, a similar number of patients referred with presumed alcohol dependence fit neither a diagnosis of dependence nor a diagnosis of abuse. Adding these together, our experience suggests that as many as one in every five patients referred for liver

Table 2.4. *Liver transplantation during alcohol dependence evaluations 1987–92*

Primary diagnosis	*n*	%
Alcohol dependence	198	74
Alcohol abuse	35	13
Other drug dependence	5	2
No diagnosis	29	11
Total	267	

transplant on the basis of suspected alcohol dependence will fail to meet the dependence criteria.

Alcohol dependence and alcoholic liver disease

For many clinicians, the presence of pathological indications of alcoholic liver disease, whether in the clinical presentation or by tissue microscopy, is synonymous with the presence of alcoholism or alcohol dependence. Consider, however, the following case history.

Case 2.1. A 37-year-old married Caucasian mother of two children was referred for transplant with signs of hepatic failure. A biopsy showed Mallory bodies and was read as alcoholic cirrhosis. At interview, she gave a negative history for alcohol dependence, corroborated by her husband and sister who were interviewed separately. Despite the team's misgivings about the discrepancy between biopsy and historical findings, she underwent transplant. She is alive and well 4 years later with no evidence of alcohol use or of non-compliance. She has been weaned from prednisone and does well on cyclosporine alone.

Alcoholic cirrhosis and alcohol dependence appear to go hand-in-hand only in about 80% of cases. As shown in Table 2.5, for example, we examined alcoholic cirrhosis as a marker for pretransplant alcohol dependence by matching those patients whom the physicians and surgeons had diagnosed as having alcoholic cirrhosis before operation against the psychiatric diagnoses taken at interview and corroborated through a family member. There was diagnostic congruity in only four of every five cases. The converse was true as well: alcohol dependence indicated a preoperative diagnosis of alcoholic cirrhosis in only three of every four cases. These figures on diagnostic agreement are very important even though tissue microscopy examination of livers removed at transplantation may offer another diagnosis. For many centers preoperative evidence for alcoholic cirrhosis forms the basis of the diagnosis on which the decision to transplant or not may reside. This is often made in the absence of a tissue diagnosis when high clinical risk contraindicates a liver biopsy. It is clear, however, that the presence of what appears to be alcoholic cirrhosis may not indicate the presence of alcohol dependence and may in fact provide a false basis from which to exclude otherwise acceptable candidates from the transplant procedure.

Screening for alcoholism

As the foregoing discussion indicates, a detailed history should be carried out as part of a proper evaluation for any transplant candidate in whom alcohol

Table 2.5. *Alcoholic cirrhosis and alcohol dependence before operation as clinical indicators of each other among liver transplant candidates*

	Cirrhosis/?dependence[a] (%)	Dependence/?cirrhosis[b] (%)
Sensitivity	95	83
Specificity	44	41
False positive	56	59
False negative	5	17
Positive predictive power	79	81
Diagnostic agreement	79	73

[a] $n = 82$.
[b] $n = 110$.

problems may be suspected. In practice an extensive evaluation, including corroboration by a family member, requires about one and one-half hours per patient. This would be impractical for the large number of patients seen in a gastroenterology or surgical clinic. Both economy and diagnostic accuracy necessitate the use of screening examinations for alcohol dependence. Research has shown that there is often a reluctance among health care personnel to address alcoholism in this setting (Geller *et al.*, 1989), especially as alcoholic patients themselves often wish to hide or minimize their condition. It is generally best to systematize screening in a way that limits these difficulties (Clark, 1981). This can be done by employing an alcohol screening examination as a routine part of the entry evaluation.

Any of several different screening examinations can be adapted for use in the general medical settings, most of which have proven to be reliable and valid when compared with the DSM-III-R diagnosis of alcohol dependence. The most brief, and therefore the most easily adapted to clinical practice, is the CAGE interview (Ewing, 1984; Table 2.6). About nine out of ten general hospital patients in the USA who answer two or more CAGE questions positively will also qualify for a diagnosis of alcohol dependence using the DSM-III-R criteria. (Beresford *et al.*, 1990) The questions are brief and may be easily worked into a routine history or physical examination. Some primary care physicians ask the questions during the physical examination in order to avoid creating a direct confrontation with the patient around questions of alcohol use.

Other screening examinations are available and may be more useful in specific settings. For example, a version of the CAGE questions, the T-ACE ques-

Table 2.6. *CAGE questions*

Have you ever felt you should Cut down on your drinking?
Have other people Annoyed you by criticizing your drinking?
Have you ever felt bad or Guilty about your drinking?
Have you ever taken a drink first thing in the morning (Eye opener) to steady your nerves or get rid of a hangover?

tions developed for use in obstetrical clinics (Sokol *et al.*, 1989), appears to be more useful when issues of guilt may carry a cultural or social stigma and may result in no response from the patient. The original screening questionnaire, the MAST (Selzer, 1971), is a pencil and paper test that can be used in an office setting. Recent research suggests that this screening examination works best for young to middle-aged males, from whom it was originally derived, and that its effectiveness is somewhat less for females or for elderly persons (Blow *et al.*, 1991).

Most clinicians would prefer to use an 'objective' indicator of alcohol dependence that is not based on the clinical history alone. Studies to date suggest that no single laboratory test will suffice for this purpose, nor will a computer construction of a series of laboratory tests (Beresford *et al.*, 1990). While abnormalities in standard laboratory parameters of nutritional status, such as the mean corpuscular volume, or of liver function, such as the transaminases, may increase a suspicion of alcoholism, altered laboratory parameters do not approach the historical screening measures in their specificity for alcoholism. The clinician should be aware of one final consideration: a positive screening test does not necessarily mean a positive diagnosis. A positive screening test is only an indication for further diagnostic interview, corroboration interview and follow-up for treatment or referral.

Diagnosis and prognosis

The prediction of future drinking patterns provides the ultimate justification for any diagnosis of alcohol dependence. The question of whether alcoholics, having apparently crossed a threshold of controlled versus uncontrolled alcohol use, can ever again engage in a predictable pattern of alcohol usage has been much debated in the largely academic war over 'controlled drinking' that buffeted the alcohol research community in the late 1970s and early 1980s. On one side were those in the treatment community and in self-help groups whose view was 'once an alcoholic, always an alcoholic'. On the other side were a series of theoreticians who believed that a resumption of controlled drinking was nearly always possible with proper attention to learning, habit formation or other factors. As evidence accrued from long-term follow-up studies of alcoholics, it became clear that resumption of controlled drinking, i.e. drinking in a regular and predictable pattern, is impossible for the vast majority of those who once lose control of their drinking habit (Polich *et al.*, 1981; Vaillant, 1983). Considering those patients with DSM-III-R alcohol dependence, including evidence of the loss-of-control phenomenon, it is clinically defensible to state that their chances of controlled alcohol use in the future, even with a new liver, is a highly unlikely event on the basis of our present knowledge (Schuckit, 1991).

Ambivalence and acceptance

Any alcohol use for an alcohol dependent person post-transplantation, must be taken as a very serious clinical sign: it is evidence of a high risk to the long-term viability of the hepatic graft. In the pretransplant evaluation this risk demands attention not only to careful diagnosis and family corroboration but also to a detailed discussion between the clinician and the patient and his family member of both the diagnosis itself and the risks involved in alcohol use post-transplantation.

When considering alcohol dependence conceptually, it is important to think both of the positive and of the negative aspects of habitual use. Most clinicians, trained in recognizing and intervening in pathological states, will have no trouble in recognizing the injurious aspects of alcohol dependence. These, after all, are well codified in the schemes noted above and in textbooks of pathology. It is often much more difficult, however, to recognize the positive aspects of alcohol use from the point of view of the alcoholic. These can include both concrete phenomena, such as staying away from the pain and discomfort of alcohol withdrawal, and very complex social effects such as an apparent change of personality or the patient's survival in an intertwined, suffocating family.

It is important that the clinician keep both the positive and the negative aspects of chronic alcohol use in mind because the dependent patient's behavior is usually very ambivalent with respect to alcohol itself. For example, a frequent problem in the clinical encounter may occur when the physician mentions some negative effect of the alcohol dependence only to have the patient speak positively of it or by some other means to indicate an unwillingness to consider stopping alcohol use or attending treatment. This is often referred to as 'denial' because of the apparent proclivity of the alcohol dependent person to ignore or deny the fact that their alcohol use has become very serious to their health or to the health of others. It is probably more precise to say that the alcoholic's reaction is one of ambivalence rather than of absolute denial. If one's view of alcohol is mixed with both pluses and minuses, an external force using the minuses to threaten the supply of alcohol or the drinking behavior leaves the alcoholic with only the recourse of holding on to the pluses at all costs (see Case 3.1). This results in a characteristic tug-of-war between patient and clinician and often leaves the clinician with a sense of frustration, if not therapeutic nihilism, when dealing with alcoholic patients. Frustration and nihilism need not be the case.

When dealing with a dependent patient whose relationship with ethyl alcohol is an ambivalent one, the clinician has the option to point out *both* the negative *and* the positive aspects of the alcohol use. By doing so, the clinician offers the alcoholic an insight into both aspects of the alcoholism as well as the assurance that the clinician can perceive both sides. At the same time, acknowledging both positives and negatives, the clinician creates an atmosphere in which the judgment of whether the alcohol use is good or bad is left up to the patient and will not be forced upon him or her. This approach is most important as only the patient can change the alcoholic behavior. To do this, the ambivalence toward alcohol use must first be resolved: it can only be resolved by the patient. The clinician can assist in a knowledgable way by pointing out alternatives both good and bad. The wise clinician will realize that he or she has no direct power to alter the drinking pattern.

From the point of view of liver transplant allocation, or when considering prognosis more generally, resolution of the alcoholic's ambivalence and a sustained effort at remaining abstinent is a necessity. For many patients requesting liver transplant, this ambivalence has already been resolved and there has been a sustained period of alcohol-free living. For others, however, the ambivalence towards drinking may persist, often in subtle ways. Perhaps the best indicator of its presence is the clinician's own sense that a particular patient has not yet come to terms with the fact that any subsequent alcohol use is a very high-risk behaviour, as in the following case.

Case 2.2. This 44-year-old Caucasian male businessman was admitted to the medical service with acute liver failure. He reported no drinking for 2 months and said he had no desire to drink. With treatment, his liver indices improved and he was discharged. He missed scheduled follow-up appointments with the internist and psychiatrist but arrived on time to see the transplant surgeon. He was jolly, cooperative and gave a plausible account of his missed medical appointments. Blood and urine screens for alcohol were positive. Confronted with this information, he remained jolly saying that he had misunderstood the internist's warnings about his liver, that he could stop drinking any time and that he had friends everywhere who could help him. Further evaluation revealed that he had alienated his family, his ex-wife and his children. He was asked to seek alcohol treatment. He did not return for further clinic visits.

Another indication may be a similar sense of discomfort among family members when considering the alcoholic person. From whatever source, the sense of discomfort is oftentimes the best clinical indicator of a referral for alcohol treatment or to a self-help support group, as the patient's physical condition will allow. In the best possible circumstance, the transplant team will be afforded sufficient time to observe the patient's course as long as possible before deciding whether to transplant.

At the same time, it is important for clinicians to understand that alcohol dependence is a treatable condition. One careful long-term study has shown that the natural remission rate for alcoholism, even among seriously debilitated alcoholics, is around 30% (Vaillant, 1983). Statistics from the literature on alcohol rehabilitation place the optimum treatment success rates in the range of 50 to 60% (Moos *et al.*, 1990). It is clear from such studies that treatment of alcoholism, beyond the acute stages of intoxication and withdrawal, is largely a treatment of hope. From other studies, it is also clear that the lack of hope results in a dismal outcome (Chafetz and Blaine, 1971). The provision of hope, the staple of the doctor/patient relationship from time immemorial, is a critical part of working with alcoholic patients who request liver transplantation. It is likewise a critical part of any successful ongoing treatment. The wise clinician, in our judgment, will tend very carefully to the sense of hope as well as to the ambivalence noted above. When this is done, recovery from alcohol use in a sustained fashion becomes itself a very hopeful exercise.

Conceptualizing alcohol dependence as a *disease* can bring hope for many patients. While most alcohol rehabilitation therapists think of alcoholism as a disease, the question of its actually being one has replaced the question of controlled drinking as the battle ground of the proprietary rehabilitation interests and some self-help groups against the theoreticians. In practice, this is largely a pointless debate. Some patients benefit from thinking of alcoholism as a disease because, in the words of one, 'It is much easier to think of myself as an ill person trying to get well than it is to think of myself as a bad person trying to be good'. On the other hand, most clinicians and therapists will have experienced an encounter with a patient who states that because alcoholism is a disease or a genetic condition visited upon them, they can do nothing about it. While there is a genetic underpinning to many forms of alcoholism

(Goodwin, 1976; Schuckit, 1991), there is no evidence that rules out choice as a factor in achieving abstinence. Choice entails hope and for many the disease concept of alcoholism provides that hope. What appears to be a substantive academic argument among those who live by academic skirmishes may only really reflect a careful clinical approach in the rehabilitation clinic, where it counts.

Non-dependent alcohol abuse

As stated above, not all patients with apparent alcoholic liver disease suffer from alcohol dependence: 13% qualify for the lesser diagnosis of alcohol abuse and another 11% fail to merit any psychiatric diagnosis (Table 2.4). Some argue that alcoholism represents a continuum of conditions and problems associated with alcohol use, whereas others define alcohol dependence as a gateway beyond which alcoholism exists and before which alarms may sound, warning of the ultimate pathology. While these views also serve as causes for theoretical extremists of one sort or another, available empirical data suggest that the presence of loss-of-control symptoms is probably the prime watershed that separates heavy drinking and addictive drinking (Vaillant, 1983; Schuckit, 1991). At the same time, there appears to be some evidence that persons who have not yet reached the stage of uncontrolled alcohol use have a better prognosis for relinquishing their drinking behavior than those for whom drinking has become an unpredictable phenomenon (Grant *et al.*, 1991). In the setting of liver transplant evaluation, we believe it is important to explore the evidence for a diagnosis of alcohol abuse that represents heavy drinking, and in this case, drinking beyond the threshold of health for one's liver, versus a state of uncontrolled addictive alcohol use. If present empirical data can be borne out with further study, it would suggest that persons who abuse alcohol and who are asked by the surgical team to abstain totally from any further alcohol use are very likely to comply and to do well over time.

Operationally, we have defined alcohol abuse in the terms suggested by the first version of the DSM-III (1980). We view alcohol abuse as the presence of mild to moderate signs of physical dependence, i.e. a developing tolerance to alcohol or occasional withdrawal symptoms from alcohol, in the absence of any symptoms of the loss-of-control phenomena and other symptoms of impaired social functioning as a result of drinking. We note that operative survival for this group, as presented in Figure 2.2, is slightly better than that for the alcohol dependent cohort, although this difference does not appear to reach statistical significance. Figure 2.2 also illustrates a remarkably poor

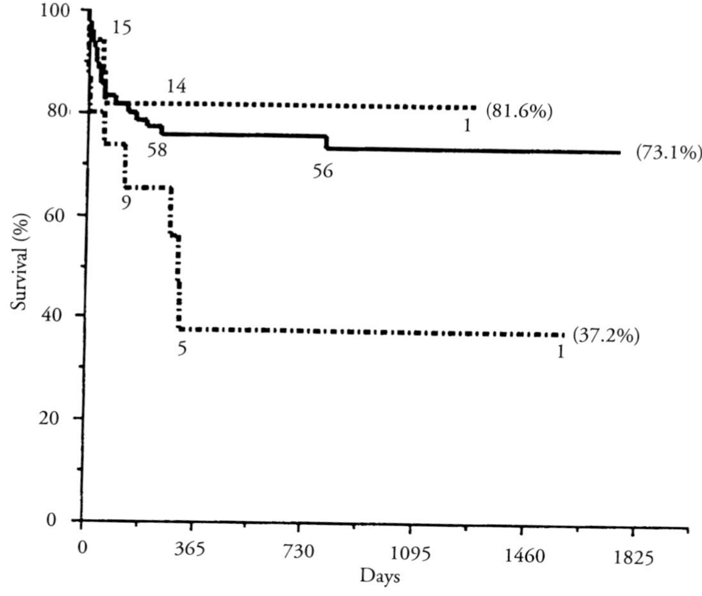

Figure 2.2. Liver transplant survival and DSM-III-R alcohol use diagnosis in 109 candidates. (–) Dependence, $n = 77$. (- - -) Abuse, $n = 17$. (- · · ·) No diagnosis.

survival outlook for suspected alcoholic patients referred to the psychiatrist but who do not merit an alcohol-related diagnosis. At the time of writing, we can only say that we are puzzled by this phenomenon and have no easily discernible explanation for it other than the relatively small numbers of cases given. We expect that for both the abusive and no-diagnosis groups, longer follow-up of larger patient samples will offer a better understanding. Whether or not, as the literature on alcohol suggests, the non-dependent alcohol abuse patients are less likely than the dependent patients to resume alcohol use after operation must also await careful follow-up studies.

Alcoholism, poly-substance abuse and severe character pathology

Prevalence estimates put the lifetime frequency of alcohol dependence at between 7% and 10% for the population of the USA (Vaillant, 1983; Schuckit, 1991). Whereas many persons make incidental use of other psychoactive substances, for the great majority of alcoholics the addictive use of ethyl alcohol serves as the primary drug of dependence. The single exception to this may be heavy nicotine use which often goes hand-in-hand with heavy drinking. There is, however, a subgroup of persons with alcohol dependence who also present a history of addiction to other substances, usually more than two, at different times in their lives. These make up approximately 0.5% of the general population and have been described as poly-substance abusers as a primary diagnostic category (Vaillant, 1988). Associated characteristics of this pattern of alcohol use generally include severe social or character problems before the age of 15 years and the use of alcohol along with other drugs during adolescence followed by heavy use through their twenties and thirties. Intravenous drug use of substances such as opiates or amphetamines, often resulting in hepatitis B or C infection, frequently occurs in this group. One may also find a high prevalence of addictive use of substances such as hallucinogens that tend to be used less commonly in the general population than are substances such as alcohol or tranquilizers. The use of stimulants such as crack cocaine or powdered cocaine may or may not be a part of this constellation depending, in part, on the availability of such substances and whether, as at the present time, an epidemic of cocaine abuse/dependence is prevalent in the general population.

The phenomenon of poly-drug abuse, including alcohol dependence, does not occur in a vacuum. The same persons may often show evidence of moderate to severe character pathology, as in the following cases.

Case 2.3. A 39-year-old divorced male gave a 22-year history of alcoholism and poly-drug dependence including intravenous use, resulting in a brief time in gaol and two failed marriages. He documented 3 years of alcohol and drug-free living. He reported attending two Alcoholics Anonymous (AA) and one Narcotics Anonymous meetings weekly and having an AA 'sponsor'. His job as a factory worker was being held for him owing to 14 years service with the same company. He noted seeing his children regularly and working with his ex-wife in caring for their youngest child who had a learning disability. He received a liver transplant, returned to work and was alive and well after 4 years.

Case 2.4. A 38-year-old female, unmarried clerk described a history of poly-drug dependence and alcoholism since mid-teens along with a history of running away from home and two vice charges. She documented having been alcohol and drug-free for the previous 4 years as well as working steadily in the same firm during this time. She attended AA only sporadically. She reported having lived with a long-time male friend for the past 3 years and was accepted as a member of his family. She received a liver transplant and was alive and well after 3 years.

Case 2.5. A 35-year-old male with alcoholic cirrhosis presented with a 17-year history of alcoholism. He also had a 15-year criminal history and was currently serving time for his third offence: armed robbery. He was not eligible for parole for another 9 years. He was married and had three young children. Prison officials could not guarantee that he would receive his postoperative medicines. He was not accepted for a graft procedure owing to concerns about his postoperative welfare.

Case 2.6. A 38-year-old divorced male was admitted to hospital with alcoholic cirrhosis and a history of intravenous drug abuse beginning in his early 20s and followed by 10 years of heavy drinking, a spotty employment history and a failed marriage. He managed to remain alcohol-free for 1 year prior to evaluation with very little social support. During the evaluation period, he was unable to follow through with a recommended diet and medicine regimen. His family stated that they were unable to 'manage him' and were ambivalent about providing further care for him. He was not accepted for transplant because of the team's concerns over his ability to manage his medicines and because of the lack of consistent social support.

Establishing a diagnosis of poly-substance abuse which may include alcoholism is vitally important from the point of view of prognosis for continued abstinence from alcohol after a liver transplant. Studies of the natural history of alcoholism in the absence of poly-substance abuse and character pathology symptoms show that pre-existing character traits do not distinguish those persons who are likely to become alcoholic from those persons who are not (Vaillant, 1983). By contrast, similar studies of persons showing character pathology in the grade school years and early adolescence are significant predictors of subsequent poly-substance abuse including alcoholism (Glueck and Glueck, 1950). For comparison, the natural remission rates for most alcoholic persons once their alcoholism has been addressed are very hopeful, generally in the range of 30–60%, depending on resources and length of follow-up in the studies presently recorded (Vaillant, 1983; Moos *et al.*, 1990). By contrast, the natural history of poly-substance addiction is often one of indurated behavior with little response to treatment until such time as the severity of both the character problems and the poly-substance abuse wanes (Vaillant, 1966). For most such persons, this generally occurs in their late 30s to early 40s. Prior to that time, some studies have suggested that the maximum rate of sustained abstinence will be no higher than 10% for this group (Vaillant, 1988).

In clinical practice, poly-substance abusers who are alcohol dependent are as likely as anyone else to suffer cirrhosis of the liver. In addition, their likelihood of suffering with hepatitis B, C or other complications resulting from chronic drug use appears to be higher than that seen in a population of persons who are dependent on alcohol alone. While in our experience we have provided liver transplants to persons with histories of poly-substance addiction and character pathology, and those patients have done well over time, we have likewise refused transplants to such persons when in our judgment the poly-addictive style of substance use had not waned. While each case must be judged on its own merits, we have generally looked to a period of 1–2 years of abstinence from poly-substances along with a reasonable social adjustment as indicators of likely postoperative abstinence and medication compliance. As in the cases noted above, relief from a poly-substance abuse style of living has often presented near the end of the fourth decade of life, as is suggested by the literature. When faced with patients of a lesser age or more pressing signs and symptoms of poly-substance abuse and characterological behavior, our approach has been to follow such patients over time in an effort to gauge whether or not they are able to refrain from the injurious use of substances and whether they are able to maintain their compliance with the prescribed regimens of medicines or diet. Here is a further case example.

Case 2.7. This 14-year-old female was transferred from another hospital with cirrhosis due to hepatitis C. She presented a 3-year history of poly- drug use including crack cocaine. She also had a history of alcohol dependence and met criteria for conduct disorder. Her father had died from alcoholic cirrhosis and her mother was unable to set behavioral limits. During a month's trial of diet and medicine regimen in hospital she demonstrated that she was unable to comply with care nand her family was unable to set limits with her sufficient to ensure her medical compliance. Psychiatric intervention with patient and family had no effect. The transplant team elected not to pursue liver graft evaluation.

When it is clear that abstinence and/or compliance are unlikely, it is difficult to pursue transplantation any further given the scarcity of donor organs. Our numbers of patients in this diagnostic category are few, however, and further experience must be accrued before our approach can be applied more generally with the confidence of statistical validity.

Alcoholism and major psychiatric disorders

There are two chronic psychiatric conditions, part of whose symptomatology includes psychosis, that may present in association with alcoholism obliging the patient and family to seek liver transplant. The first is schizophrenia, which occurs in about 1% of the population in the USA, and the second is the affective disorder of depression and mania, which affects approximately 4% of the population of the USA. Persons suffering any of these major psychiatric disorders have a considerably higher risk of developing alcohol dependence than do persons in the general population. In schizophrenia, for example, the risk is estimated to be two to three times greater than for the general population (Pulver *et al.*, 1989). Clinical study also suggests that even minimal drinking in schizophrenic patients can result in exacerbations of this debilitating condition (Drake *et al.*, 1989). The major psychiatric disorders are chronic conditions and the issues of continued compliance with postoperative medications become salient even though we have effective medicines with which to manage these conditions for the great majority of those suffering from them.

Transplant candidates presenting with major psychiatric disorders in addition to alcoholism must be evaluated carefully with respect to the extent, the duration and the previous results of treatment. While there is no evidence to suggest that any of these conditions must constitute an absolute contraindication to liver transplant, the presence of a chronic psychotic illness along with alcohol dependence is generally regarded as a troubling prognostic sign. It is important for the clinician to note, however, that there is a wide individual variation in the presentation and course of each of these disorders and that this must be explored for decision making purposes. While surveys of transplant teams show that most programs take psychiatric comorbidity into account (Olbrisch and Levenson, 1991), no sizeable case series details either experience with persons suffering from the major psychiatric disorders or their course after transplantation. In the absence of such detail, standard guidelines of medical care of persons with major psychoses must be considered in this clinical decision.

We have listed in Table 2.7 these and other psychiatric conditions that may potentially rule out the liver graft procedure. Those that we have not mentioned in this chapter are rarely seen in liver transplant candidates with the exception of dementing illness. Cognitive impairment frequently occurs among transplant candidates, generally due to hepatic encephalopathy resulting from hyperammonemic states. While these can be subtle or pronounced, they usually respond to proper medical therapy, are nearly always reversible and therefore resemble delirious processes rather than dementing illness (see Chapter 3). Irreversible dementias, by contrast, are seen infrequently among those applying to tertiary care centers for liver transplant. The most common dementia, Alzheimer's disease, generally manifests itself to primary clinicians and contraindicates transplantation because of its irreversibilty.

Of special importance among alcoholics is the Wernicke–Korsakoff syndrome, especially Korsakoff's "psychosis" which must include a clear loss of recent memory function and may include a global confusional state in the worst cases. Consistent with the published literature (Victor *et al.*, 1971), the Wernick–Korsakoff syndrome also occurs relatively infrequently in transplant candidates. We have seen one case.

Table 2.7. *Possible psychiatric contraindications to liver transplant*

Major psychiatric disorders
Schizophrenia
Affective illness
Depression
Mania
Anxiety disorders
Obsessive compulsive disorder
Alcoholism
Poly-drug abuse
Character disorders
Sociopathy
Borderline/narcissistic disorders
Hysteria/Briquet syndrome
Irreversible dementias
Alzheimer's disease
Wernicke–Korsakoff syndrome
Alcoholic dementia

Case 2.8. A 38-year-old man with a profound short-term memory disorder, a very unstable social situation and a history of 20 years of heavy drinking was referred for evaluation. There was no nystagmus or ophthalmoplegia. There was no gait disturbance although the finger-nose test suggested mild cerebellar impairment. His cognitive functions were otherwise clear with some lack of concentration when subtracting serial sevens. His ammonia level was within the normal range. The team elected to follow him for 6 months by which time his memory had improved only minimally and his social situation not at all. The team decided against offering a transplant because his memory impairment had been only partly reversible, casting much doubt on his ability to care for himself.

Most of such cases are not referred for transplant because of the irreversibility of the cognitive impairment, an absolute contraindication in most programs. As this case demonstrates, the Korsakoff syndrome can be diagnosed only when presumed hepatic encephalopathy or other apparent deliria have been treated. The question of reversibility must then be assessed with adequate follow-up evaluation including assurance of adequate nutrition and abstinence from alcohol.

Another relatively infrequent syndrome, alcoholic dementia, may present in a similar manner and must be differentiated from both hepatic encephalopathy and the Korsakoff syndrome. Alcoholic dementia is a poorly defined entity in which a patient may present with a global cognitive impairment, in contrast to the selective impairments seen in early cases of Alzheimer's disease, but an intact recent memory ability inconsistent with the Korsakoff syndrome. The global impairment of cognition in association with many years of heavy drinking constitutes this syndrome; recent data suggest that the presence of an associated peripheral neuropathy, ataxia, coarse nystagmus and a lack of anomia are particularly useful tests in evaluating patients for this condition (R.M Atkinson, personal communication). While its occurrence as a condition distinct from the Wernicke–Korsakoff syndrome is a matter of controversy, a transplant candidate presenting with a suspected history of alcoholic dementia should receive a careful dementia evaluation along with appropriate neuropsychologic testing before the diagnosis can be made.

Role of the psychiatrist on the transplant team

The make-up and functioning of transplant teams vary greatly from one instit-ution to another. Studies of various approaches have begun to appear in the literature but these for the most part document inclusion and exclusion criteria rather than the exact roles of specific persons in the decision making process (Olbrisch and Levenson, 1991). To the best of our knowledge, however, it is not the role of the psychiatrist to decide on inclusion or exclusion of a patient for liver transplant. Final decisions appear to be made in one of two ways: either through a triage model in which the most senior surgeon makes the final decision after having reviewed all of the information from a multidisciplinary evaluation or through a committee model in which a consensus de-cision is arrived at after a similar review of all the available information. In either of these models, however, the psychiatrist's role is that of a consultant who provides a specialized evaluation, a psychiatric diagnosis when one is merited, and a statement of the likelihood of prognosis for long-term abstinence or good outcome. As may be gathered from the discussion thus far, the diagnostic statement is perhaps the most clearly defined while the statements of prognosis tend to be much less precise. This fact may be irritating to some who might prefer an unequivocal statement about the future course.

Unfortunately, present knowledge of the course and prediction of recovery from alcoholism simply cannot sustain any but qualified statements. In extreme 'high-risk' cases, such as those with very little or no social support, no recognition of an underlying alcohol problem, no hope for the future and no resources to manage continued abstinence, the psychiatric opinion may be less equivocal than for most such cases. The same may obtain for persons at the other end of the spectrum, those who have had some episode of alcohol dependent behavior but who have managed long-term abstinence with all of the prognostic factors noted above. The prime difficulty comes for the large group of alcoholic patients between these extremes who manifest some good prognostic factors but not all. In such cases, the psychiatrist will most likely offer a qualified opinion and request further opinions by different observers at different points in time as a way of improving on the original impression. Alcohol dependence is a long-term illness. Continued follow-up is most often necessary and will most likely increase the levels both of certainty and of comfort that the clinical team may require in deciding on cases that are not clearly included or excluded from consideration.

References

The Diagnostic and Statistical Manual, (1980). 3rd edn. Washington, DC, American Psychiatric Association.

The Diagnostic and Statistical Manual, (1987). 3rd edn., revised. Washington, DC, American Psychiatric Association.

Atkinson, R. M. (1990). Aging and alcohol use disorders: diagnostic issues in the elderly. *International Psychogeriatrics*, **2**, 55–72.

Beresford, T. P., Blow, F.C., Hill, E.M., and Singer, K. (1991). When is an alcoholic an alcoholic? *Alcohol and Alcoholism*, **26** (Suppl. 1), 487–8.

Beresford, T. P., Blow, F. C., Hill, E., Singer, K. and Lucey, M. R. (1990). Comparison of CAGE questionnaire and computer-assisted laboratory profiles in screening for covert alcoholism. *Lancet*, **336**, 482–5.

Blow, F. C., Brower, K.J., Young, J.P., Hill, E.M., Singer, K.M. and Beresford, T.P. (1991). Predictive value of brief alcoholism screening tests in a sample of hospitalized adults. *Alcoholism: Clinical and Experimental Research*, **15**, 374.

Cahalan, D. (1970). *Problem Drinkers: a National Survey*. San Francisco, Jossey–Bass.

Chafetz, M.E. and Blaine, H.T. 1971. *Frontiers Of Alcoholism*. New York, Science House.

Clark, W. D. (1981). Alcoholism: blocks to diagnosis and treatment. *American Journal of Medicine*, **71**, 275–86.

Drake, R.E., Osher, F.C. and Wallach, M.A. (1989). Alcohol use and abuse in schizophrenia. A prospective community study. *Journal of Nervous and Mental Disease*,**177**, 408–14

Ewing, J. A. (1984). Detecting alcoholism: the CAGE questionnaire. *Journal of the American Medical Association*, **252**, 1905–7.

Geller, G. L., Levine, D.M., Mammon, J.A., Moore, R.D., Bone, L.R. and Stokes, E.J. (1989). Knowledge, attitudes and reported practices of medical students and house staff regarding the diagnosis and treatment of alcoholism. *Journal of the American Medical Association*, **261**, 3115–20.

Glueck, S. and Glueck, E. (1950). *Unravelling Juvenile Delinquency*. New York, The Commonwealth Fund.

Goodwin, D.W. (1976). *Is Alcoholism Hereditary?* New York, Oxford University Press.

Grant, B., DeBakey, S and Zobeck, TS. (1991). *Liver Cirrhosis Mortality In the United States, Surveillance Report* no. 18 . Washington, DC, US Department of Health and Human Services.

Moos, R. M., Finney, J.W. and Cronkite, R.C. (1990). *Alcoholism Treatment.* New York, Oxford University Press.

Olbrisch, M. E. and Levenson, J. L. (1991). Psychosocial evaluation of heart transplant candidates: an international survey of process, criteria, and outcomes. *Journal of Heart and Lung Transplantation,* **10**, 948–55.

Polich, J. M., Armor, D.J. and Braker, H.B. (1981). *The Course Of Alcoholism: Four Years After Treatment*. New York, Wiley.

Pulver, A.E., Wolyniec, P.S., Wagner, M.G., Moorman, C.C. and McGrath, J.A. (1989). An epidemiologic investigation of alcohol-dependent schizophrenics. *Acta Psychiatrica Scandinavia,* **79**, 603–12.

Schuckit, M. A. (1991). *Drug and Alcohol Abuse, A Clinical Guide To Diagnosis and Treatment* 3rd edn. New York, Plenum Press.

Selzer, M. L. (1971). The Michigan alcoholism screening test: the quest for a new diagnostic instrument. *American Journal of Psychiatry,* **127**, 1653–8.

Sokol, R. J., Martier, S. S. and Ager, J. W. (1989). The T-ACE questions: practical prenatal detection of risk-drinking (see comments). *American Journal of Obstetrics and Gynecology,* **160**, 863–8.

Surman, O.S. (1989). Psychiatric aspect of organ transplantation. *American Journal of Psychiatry,* **146**, 972–82.

Vaillant, G.E. (1966). A twelve-year follow-up of New York narcotic addicts. IV. *American Journal of Psychiatry,* **123**, 573–84.

Vaillant, G.E. (1983). *The Natural History Of Alcoholism.* Cambridge, MA, Harvard University Press.

Vaillant, G.E. (1988). The alcohol-dependent and drug-dependent person. In *The New Harvard Guide To Psychiatry,* ed. A.M. Nicholi. Cambridge, Harvard University Press.

Victor, M., Adams, R.D. and Collins, G.H. (1971). *The Wenicke–Korsakoff Syndrome.* Philadelphia, F. A. Davis.

Zakim, D., Boyer, T.D. and Montgomery, C. (1989). Alcoholic liver disease. In *Hepatology , A Textbook of Liver Disease,* 2nd edn, eds B. Zakim and T.D. Boyer, pp. 821–62). Philadelphia, W.B. Saunders.

CHAPTER THREE

PSYCHIATRIC ASSESSMENT OF ALCOHOLIC CANDIDATES FOR LIVER TRANSPLANTATION

THOMAS P. BERESFORD

Introduction

It is one thing to view alcoholism and liver disease from the perspective of epidemiology or cell biology and another to bring this knowledge to bear on the clinical situation. In the case of liver transplantation, in which there is a scarcity of liver grafts and no equally effective alternative therapy, the transplant team must make judgments in good faith on the likelihood of every candidate's ability to preserve the functioning of the grafted liver after the operation. This is nowhere more difficult than in assessing the likelihood that an alcoholic liver transplant recipient will refrain from the behavior that resulted in the demise of his or her native liver. Our transplant team and others have faced this task and there is a nascent body of systematically collected experience on the topic (Beresford *et al.*, 1990; Bird *et al.*, 1990;Kumar, *et al.*, 1990; Lucey *et al.*, 1992; Mentha *et al.*, 1991; Mirza *et al.*, 1991; Starzl *et al.*, 1988). This chapter reviews current methods of patient selection including the data accumulated over the past 6 years. We discuss alternative approaches to selection used in different transplant centers and offer critical views in the hope of improving the process. In Chapter 6, what is known about post-transplant outcome among alcoholic recipients is discussed.

The drinking history

In Chapter 2 the importance of providing a diagnosis of alcohol dependence or establishing its absence was discussed. Once a diagnosis is established, as it is in the great majority of patients referred for alcohol use evaluation, the clinician must use this information to assist the patient towards seeking help. In one approach, for example, the clinician reviews each patient's alcohol use history with that patient and again with both the patient and a family member together. This serves two purposes: to review the basis for assigning a diagnosis of alcohol dependence including the risk of future drinking behavior and to offer the clinician an opportunity to observe how both the patient and the family member accept this diagnosis as an important part of the health history. The patient's recognition of uncontrolled alcohol use as a problem that has to be faced is the essential first step in further care. In our experience, and in that of others, patients who are unable to recognize their alcohol problem should not be considered further for their transplant as exemplified in the following case.

Case 3.1. This 59-year-old Caucasian divorced woman lived with her son and his family. He described her as having usually drunk one fifth gallon of scotch daily, with regular withdrawal symptoms, for many years until she had learned of her liver failure 3 months earlier. Her son described her as isolated from the family because of their insistence that she seek treatment for alcoholism and because they could no longer tolerate her drinking when working in the family business. She stated that she was not an alcoholic but that she would give up drinking until her liver was better. The transplant team did not continue the evaluation beyond that point.

This case illustrates what is commonly called 'denial' of the alcoholism: a patient refusing to acknowledge a problem despite overwhelming evidence to the contrary. Note, however, that the patient's son emphasizes only the negative aspects of his mother's drinking. To those who work with alcoholic cases the term 'denial' may sound too simplistic. For most alcoholics, the relation-

Table 3.1. *Physician/patient agreement on alcohol dependence diagnosis*

Diagnosis	*n*	%
Agree	190	81.5
Disagree	43	18.5

ship with alcohol is not one of exclusive attention but of ambivalence, often an intensely felt ambivalence. Each time an outside force attempts to remove the alcohol, the patient is left only with one choice: to hold on to the drinking as tightly as possible.

A more effective approach with most alcoholics is to articulate *both* sides of the ambivalence and to leave the decision on whether to drink or not in the patient's hands (see Chapter 2). This approach requires the clinician to elicit and then to appreciate the positive aspects of the drinking from the patient's point of view: 'Alcohol quells some of my anxieties even though it causes others; it is a comforting habit; it is available at any time; it keeps me away from withdrawal,' and so on. In the words of one alcoholic who found his way to long-term sobriety, 'It was like an abusive lover. I knew it was bad for me but I didn't want to give it up. I finally had to decide for myself not to drink'. It is often the case that in our zeal to identify and treat the pathology of drinking we over emphasize the negative aspects of chronic, uncontrolled alcohol use when attention to both positive and negative effects would be more appropriate.

Table 3.1 lists the frequencies of agreement between clinician and patient in 233 cases of alcohol dependence or abuse gleaned from the patient's own clinical history. In the majority of cases, the patient agreed with the diagnosis and indicated an understanding of the risks of subsequent drinking. For one case in five, however, this was not true. The clinician must be careful to document the clinical history and diagnostic impressions as they may serve as a primary reason for refusing transplantation. In this circumstance, it is best that the patient be seen by more than one observer and preferably at different points in time. In this way, the original clinical impression can be independently assessed and either corroborated or discarded.

A minority of those in the alcoholism research community may argue that 'diagnosis' in and of itself is valueless and that no one should be required to 'agree' with any clinical perception (Makela and Room, 1985). This is counterbalanced by the necessity of defining a clear syndrome that both the patient and the physician may follow in ongoing care. And it is substantiated by prospective, longitudinal data that leaves little doubt as to the natural course of active, recognizable alcoholism (Polich *et al.*, 1981; Vaillant, 1983).

Taking the pledge

Some programs in the USA will ask the patient to sign a 'contract' or a pledge in which they clearly state that they understand the seriousness of their drinking history, the fact of its being a chronic risk, and their intention to continue to abstain from alcohol after the transplant for the rest of their life. While on the surface this may seem an unrealistic exercise given the small impact of motivation at one point in time to produce long-term abstinence, those programs using this technique point out that this method documents, prior to the transplant, both the patient's recognition of their alcoholism and their understanding of the need to remain abstinent. According to those who use this approach, if drinking relapse were to occur after transplant the clinician is poised to provide care aided by this earlier documentation of the problem.

Our experience on this issue has been mixed. On the one hand, we have noted patients who were clearly alcohol dependent, who agreed with their clinician's perception of their dependence before transplant but 6 or 12 months after transplant reported that they no longer suffered from alcohol dependence or that drinking was a risk for them (Beresford *et al.*, 1992). It is difficult to know whether signing an agreement of this nature would have made any difference this perception. Similarly, we have noted that non-alcoholic transplant recipients, even though advised by the transplant team not to drink any alcohol after the surgery, frequently resumed social drinking (see Chapter 6). While understanding the rationale of using a 'contract', we consider its practical value is limited. Our approach, rather, has been to provide follow-up visits at regular intervals during which sobriety and continuing motivation can be assessed. This reflects the view that the ongoing contact and commitment probably weigh more heavily in the service of abstinence than does a one-time written agreement.

Length of preoperative sobriety

Early on, many transplant centers required a preset period of sobriety by the candidate as a requirement for a liver graft. Lengths of required sober time were as long as 1 year in some centers. In the USA, such requirements have been gradually shortened partly as a result of a court case in which the judge

Table 3.2. *Preoperative length of sobriety*

		Length of sobriety	
	n	>6 months *n* (%)	<6 months *n* (%)
Alcohol dependence	198	105 (53)	93 (47)
Alcohol abuse	35	16 (46)	19 (54)

held that the length of sobriety could not reasonably be longer than the natural course of the alcoholic cirrhosis itself (Beresford, *et al.*, 1990). Today, some programs still require a period of sobriety of 3–6 months before providing a liver transplant.

In our early experience, we noted that there seemed to be little relationship between the length of preoperative abstinence from alcohol and subsequent survival of the transplant procedure (Beresford, *et al.*, 1990). Further experience (Table 3.2) with a larger number of patients has confirmed this. Half of the alcohol dependent and abusive patients referred for evaluation have abstained for 6 months or less at the time of transplant with no evident difference in transplant survival rates compared with those who have abstained for longer periods. Another group has noted informally that transplant patients who were sober less than 6 months used more hospital resources during the preoperative period than did those whose abstinence was greater than 6 months. An analysis of data on resource utilization from our program did not corroborate this (McCurry *et al.*, 1992). The most important clinical question is whether or not the length of preoperative sobriety predicts the length of postoperative sobriety for alcohol dependent transplant recipients. At present the numbers of alcoholic liver graft recipients who then proceeded to imbibe alcohol are too small to make reasonable comparisons. This question must await longer follow-up, probably through a multicenter study, to provide sound empirical data.

Preoperative encephalopathy

Table 3.3 illustrates the frequency of hepatic encephalopathy in a large series of patients referred for alcohol use evaluation. About one-third of patients seeking liver transplantation present with at least one previous episode of hepatic encephalopathy, i.e. episodic confusion reversed with medical treatment of the

Table 3.3. *Hepatic encephalopathy at evaluation*

	n	%
History of encephalopathy	95	35.3
Mini-Mental State (*n* = < 23)	19	7.1

Total patients evaluated = 269.

hyperammonemia. Many more patients had shorter episodes of transient memory impairment or other mild cognitive dysfunction from the same cause. At the time of the psychiatrist's interview, about 7% of the total number of patients presented with florid cognitive impairment as measured by the Hopkins Mini-Mental State Examination (Folstein *et al.*, 1975), a careful examination of mental status at the time of evaluation. While studies have documented pervasive neuropsychological deficits on specialized testing (Trzepacz *et al.*, 1989; Arria *et al.*, 1991), for many alcoholic transplant candidates in the clinical encounter, attention to tests of recent memory and of judgment is especially important. An alcoholic patient with mild encephalopathy may appear as one who has not overcome their alcohol dependence, causing the clinician to refer the patient for alcohol treatment. In most instances, this course is not justified because the attention and memory impairment make alcohol rehabilitation impractical as it depends heavily on the patient's learning capacities for success. Similarly, standard questions involving judgment in hypothetical situations may reveal the lack of an adequate understanding of the transplant procedure and compliance with postoperative medication. Both areas should be reassessed after medical treatment of the encephalopathy. Further differentiation of the causes of cognitive dysfunction are discussed in Chapters 2 and 6.

Factors in standard questioning involving both memory and compliance can be used to establish the mental competency of the candidate to accept a liver transplant procedure. This requires the interviewer to assess whether the patient understands the nature of a liver transplant and can describe it in his or her own words, whether they understand the likely consequences of treatment of their liver disease with a transplant and whether they understand the consequence of no treatment of their liver disease. In the great majority of cases, patients will be able to explain these contingencies clearly. In some cases, however, encephalopathy prevents this and must be treated as effectively as possible before proceeding with the transplant evaluation.

Table 3.4. *Strauss–Bacon social stability scale*

Characteristic	Point score
Steady job for the past three years	1
Same residence for the past two years	1
Married and lives with spouse	1
Does not live alone	1

Table 3.5. *Preoperative social stability score*

	Social stability score		
Alcohol	*n*	2 or less *n* (%)	3 or more *n* (%)
Dependence	198	66 (33)	132 (67)
Abuse	35	4 (11)	31 (89)

Social stability

The stereotypic caricature of an alcoholic portrays a resident of 'Skid Row': living on the streets, alone and with no means of support. It is important to remember that this is indeed a stereotype, that only a very small minority of alcoholics in the USA fit this description (Vaillant, 1983; Schuckit, 1991). The vast majority have a stable residence, maintain contact with their families and have a means of earning a living. Nevertheless, when considering a liver graft procedure followed by a lifetime of anti-immune medicines, social stability must be assessed because it affects both long-term remission from alcoholism and compliance with an often complicated medical regimen. Strauss and Bacon (1951) noticed long ago that a socially stable adjustment was associated with continued participation in alcohol treatment. In their study, persons presenting with three or more of the four characteristics presented in Table 3.4 were likely to remain in treatment. As noted in Table 3.5, most of our patients meet this criterion. Other programs use similar indices of social stability (Skinner *et al.*, 1981).

One limitation of this scale is its weighting towards employment outside the home, a factor that may apply more frequently to the preponderantly male population of alcoholics rather than to females. In using the Strauss–Bacon

Table 3.6. *Negative prognostic factors*

Pre-existing psychotic disorder
Unstable character disorder
Unremitted poly-drug abuse
Multiple alcohol rehabilitation attempts
Social isolation

scale, we include homemaking or child rearing as evidence of gainful employment in an attempt to apply this scale equally to both sexes. Another limitation will be obvious to experienced clinicians: there is a wide range of individual variability in the areas of functioning assessed by the Strauss–Bacon scale. These data, therefore, must always be used in the context of the specific case history as well as the corroborating family discussion. Even in the instance of a patient who scores two or less on the Strauss-Bacon scale, the social stability criteria remain only one part of the overall evaluation, as discussed elsewhere in this chapter.

Abstinence: negative prognostic factors

Researchers have noted other factors which, when present, can be associated with a return to drinking (Table 3.6) Social isolation or instability is often seen in association with other phenomena, such as chronic mental illness. These phenomena generally include psychotic states, such as the major affective disorders, in both the depressed and the manic forms, as well as schizophrenia. Present knowledge suggests that the combination of a chronic psychosis and the existence of alcohol dependence worsens the likelihood of stable, long-term abstinence (see Chapter 2) while lesser conditions, such as the anxiety disorders, may also predispose towards alcohol addiction if alcohol use to treat the anxiety leads to dependence. At the same time, the presence of a major mental illness greatly increases the likelihood of concurrent alcohol or other substance dependence. In such instances, therefore, the clinician must assess both previous alcohol and drug usage and the psychiatric history.

The co-occurrence of a major psychiatric disorder does not serve as an absolute contraindication for transplant but, the patient and the transplant team will be more dependent on the patient's social support network to ensure continued compliance and to warn about resumed drinking than would be the case in a patient without a major psychiatric disorder. In our experience, and that of others, such cases have been relatively rare. An increased clinical knowledge of the assessment of such cases must await multicenter studies in which sufficient numbers of appropriate subjects will give a meaningful analysis.

A more troubling negative prognostic factor exists in the patient who clearly acknowledges alcohol dependence and whose family corroborates it but whose history is one of 'revolving door' treatment experiences followed by limited periods of continued abstinence. In some studies, frequent attempts at alcohol treatment have been viewed as indicators of a poor ultimate prognosis (Smith and Cloninger, 1985). Vaillant and colleagues in a prospective longitudinal study (Vaillant, 1983; Valliant *et al.*, 1983) reached the opposite conclusion: that the number of times a person attended an Alcoholics Anonymous (AA) meeting was highly correlated with the existence of stable long-term (greater than three years) abstinence. In general, patients who present with multiple unsuccessful attempts at alcohol rehabilitation, whether through clinics, support groups or other means, must be assessed carefully for other factors militating for a good outcome that might counterbalance these previous experiences. At the same time, the clinician must recall the fact that the drinking patient's ambivalence toward alcohol must be resolved before stable abstinence can follow, no matter how often treatment exposure has occurred. This can be a lengthy process as is evident in the following case.

Case 3.2. This 34-year-old married woman was warned of her liver disease 5 years before transplant evaluation. She attended an alcoholic rehabilitation program 1 year later but resumed drinking in a few months. She attended a second rehabilitation program 3 years before the evaluation, commenting 'I was beginning to stay dry for myself, not for everyone else'. She abstained for only another 6 months. Eighteen months before transplant evaluation she had her last drink and began attending AA meetings two to three times weekly. At evaluation, she presented a history of two failed rehabilitation attempts that were counterbalanced by her abstinence, a history corroborated by her husband.

When it is medically possible, referral to an alcohol rehabilitation program or a self-help group may give the candidate a direct experience of the likelihood of continued abstinence from alcohol. This can allow direct observation of the candidate's abstinence and may lead to improvement in the liver status that results from longer periods of observation pretransplant. Nonetheless, the prognostic case of the 'revolving door alcoholic' who possesses significant resources for recovery remains a difficult question for clinical research.

Abstinence: positive prognostic factors

When assessing candidates for liver transplantation it is not sufficient to note only those factors that are highly associated with a return to drinking. The clinician must at the same time evaluate those factors that are conducive to abstinence and to long-term health. On the basis of longitudinal, prospective research, Vaillant (1983) proposed four factors that were associated with continued long-term abstinence from alcohol: (1) substitute dependency, (2) rehabilitation relationship, (3) source of hope or renewed self-esteem, and (4) negative consequence of drinking. The presence of any two of these factors indicated a high likelihood of abstinence for 3 years or more. When only one or none of the factors was present, the likelihood of abstinence was significantly less, with a maximum of 2 years abstinence.

The first factor was the presence of an activity, 'a substitute dependency' in Vaillant's terms, with which the alcoholic replaced unstructured drinking time with structured activities that did not involve drinking. This can mean any of a series of activities ranging from a renewed interest in work or family through participation in self-help groups and volunteer or recreational activities. In its essence, this factor requires frequent participation in the activity for long periods of time. The rationale derives from the alcohol dependent person's point of view: for many drinking has been a pleasurable, self-reinforcing pastime. It is very easy to resume drinking unless some replacement is found for the behavior that has occupied a large part of one's life. In practice, many persons presenting with end-stage liver failure are physically too ill to participate immediately in such activities before the transplant. It is important, however, in those persons who have had extended abstinence periods in the past, that the clinician document the use made of the periods of abstinence and the resources that are available now to limit the amount of 'dead' time that may serve as a prelude to drinking.

The second of Vaillant's factors is the presence of a rehabilitation relationship: a person in the drinker's life who unambivalently signals their belief in the human worth of the alcohol dependent person while at the same time unambivalently imposes a limit on the drinking behavior. This person must give the clear message that the drinking person can stay but that the drinking itself must go. Many people can serve this purpose: a spouse who has worked through the difficulties caused by the alcoholic drinking in the first place, a knowledgeable friend, a professional therapist or counsellor, a sponsor from Alcoholics Anonymous, a minister, or a number of other possible people who are important in the alcohol dependent person's life.

Over the short term, the staff of the transplant team serve this same purpose: they clearly signal their belief in the worth of their alcoholic patient when they give him or her a liver graft. At the same time, most programs make it clear that drinking after the operation must be avoided to preserve the functioning of the graft. This provides an essential focus: the responsibility for abstinence behavior rests with and only with the dependent person. To abstain or to drink is a decision that only the alcohol dependent person can make. Consequently, significant others, including the transplant team members, will avoid struggles over drinking, will call for professional help should drinking resume and will be prepared to draw behavioral limits when indicated.

In operational terms, each alcohol dependent transplant candidate must demonstrate at least the presence of a 'safety valve' person who can alert the transplant team if drinking behavior resumes. In that instance, the team can present treatment alternatives and take an active role in offering alcohol rehabilitation. It is useful, when interviewing a family member in the presence of the alcohol dependent candidate, for the clinician to ask a question along the following lines: 'If, a year after the operation, Mr X begins to talk about the possibility of drinking or indeed says that he has been drinking, what would be your response?' Clinician, patient and family member (or significant other person) may then work through a plan whereby local resources come into play or the patient returns to the transplant center. The purpose of this exercise is to assure the team that a safety person exists in the candidate's life who will call for help if needed. It is to assure both the patient and the significant other person that professional help is available and should be utilized as quickly as possible should drinking relapse occur. The clinician may wish to review the two medical justifications for this with the candidate and the family member: (1) that the effect of alcohol, especially in large amounts, on a transplanted liver is not well understood and may represent a significant medical danger, and (2) that the re-establishment of continued drinking often brings with it an inattention to compliance with anti-immune medications. If the latter were to occur followed by the start of a rejection episode, dire medical consequences are likely to ensue, including liver failure and death.

Often, when the clinician raises the possibility of future drinking, both patient and spouse will protest that the drinking person intends never to drink again. The clinician will listen politely to these words and respond by saying that the question itself does not imply that the person will or will not drink again but only looks to a method of assuring the long-term health and functioning of the patient and his graft. This reflects a necessary reality: neither the clinician nor the alcoholic can be entirely certain of the alcohol dependent patient's future drinking behavior. The only useful certainty lies in the consecutive days of abstinence in the immediate past. This kind of certainty is often best accrued 'one day at a time', to use the words of Alcoholics Anonymous.

Vaillant's third factor involves finding a source of improved hope and self-esteem in the drinking person's life that can be used in the service of abstinence. It is important to recall that for most alcohol dependent persons, the drinking, whether for reasons relating to the impaired control phenomenon, to social consequences, to the physical consequences of liver damage or to some combination of these, often leads to a profound sense of guilt in the drinking person. Often in response to this guilt, the drinker may begin taking steps to hide the drinking behavior itself. As mentioned in Chapter 2, direct questions about drinking alcohol often trigger the sense of guilt and result in less than straightforward answers. From the point of view of abstinence, recurring thoughts of guilt over one's past behavior or its results can of themselves provide a significant impetus for resuming drinking. Alcoholics Anonymous has a term for this: the Poor Me's. 'Poor me. Pour me a drink!' A powerful antidote to the guilt-to-drinking procession is a counterbalancing sense of hope or self-esteem established in the alcoholic's life that can make this post-drinking sense of guilt ineffective as a factor in promoting drinking. At the the same time it may provide a useful perspective in the way of healing past injuries through one's present behavior. As Vaillant points out, the process of doing good for others is a powerful source of self-esteem.

Operationally, improved hope and self-esteem can be found in activities that promote abstinence, such as participation in a self-help group. But there are many other possibilities that might include participating in one's religion with a renewed sense of belonging, renewing hope for the future through contact with one's children or grandchildren or helping others who are about to undergo transplant by participation in a support group, to name only a few possible options. At interview, the clinician might ask questions such as, 'What keeps you going in the face of your illness or the misfortunes caused by your drinking?' 'If you find yourself feeling guilty about things that resulted from your drinking, what can you do to make those feelings better?' 'Are there any areas in your life which you consider spiritual or in which you find a sense of solace from the troubles of daily living?' Of the factors that Vaillant outlines, this is probably the most difficult to assess in a quantifiable manner. Nonetheless, as others have pointed out (Frank, 1991), the sense of hope and looking positively toward the future is of crucial importance in not only maintaining abstinence but in approaching a significant event in one's life such as surgery of this magnitude.

Vaillant's final factor involves a direct, negative behavioral consequence of the drinking. Specifically this refers to a noxious event that will happen with certainty each and every time the person imbibes alcohol. Very few conse-

Table 3.7. *Frequencies of Vaillant's prognostic factors before surgery in 198 alcohol dependent candidates*

	n	%
Substitute activities	84	42
Source of improved hope/self-esteem	127	64
Rehabilitation relationship	156	79
Negative consequence from drinking	7	4

quences of chronic drinking fulfill the requirements. Some that do include acute pancreatic pain, returning to jail for violation of parole, or the ethanol-disulfiram reaction. Liver failure itself rarely provides a potent negative consequence because of the subtlety and chronicity of its symptoms. The same is true for other physical derangements such as alcohol-induced cardiomyopathy or nerve damage. The loss of spouse or family may sometimes fit into this category depending on the firmness of their ability to set limits in the face of renewed drinking.

In operational terms, there are few negative occurrences before the transplant itself, as demonstrated in Table 3.7. The first three of Vaillant's factors are relatively frequent both before and after operation but after transplant there is a distinct perception among alcoholic patients that a noxious event, namely death, will happen to them should their drinking recur (see Table 6.2). This appears to be part of the rigor of the physical insult of the operation itself but may also result from the transplant team's preoperative instruction on the cause of liver failure and the likelihood of further complications if drinking does not cease.

In a later paper (Vaillant, 1988), Vaillant commented that the essence of all these prognostic factors is to provide structure in the life of an alcohol dependent person where no structure existed before, largely because of the inordinately large amounts of time and energy spent either in drinking or in recovering from the effects of drinking. It is a short leap to suggest that most structured uses of the patient's time will militate towards long-term abstinence. When following transplant patients after the operation, it is important that the team pay attention to each of these factors and not rely on any one of them to carry the total weight of abstinence itself. Two or more of the four factors present means that the person has begun to make significant changes in his or her life and, as a rule, efforts on all four fronts are very useful. In giving us these factors, Vaillant has provided a common map of the seemingly many pathways to long-term abstinence. It is the task of the clinicians of the transplant team to assist their patients in devising their own personal maps and then following them.

Can the clinician be sure?

When transplant teams must rely on clinical and corroborating histories as the best indicators of drinking behavior, the possibility of patients or family members providing false information always exists, as occurred in the following instance, the only one to the best of our knowledge out of 300 alcohol dependent patients evaluated and of nearly 100 transplanted:

Case 3.3. A 35-year-old mother of two children, aged 8 and 9 years, was referred from an outlying district for evaluation of liver failure due to alcohol use. During evaluation, she stated on repeated occasions to many of the team personnel, as well as to the psychiatrist, that her drinking was 'social', no more than one or two cans of beer monthly and occasional glasses of wine at the Christmas holidays. She cited her impoverished circumstances as the reason for not wasting money on alcohol. Despite the transplant team's request her husband said he was unable to participate in person in an interview. He agreed to a phone interview during which he denied that alcohol use had ever been a problem for his wife or, on specific questioning, for himself.

Seven months after transplant, the patient was admitted to hospital for liver failure. Her blood alcohol level was 120 mg/dl but was not accompanied by signs of intoxication. Biopsy of her liver was consistent with alcoholic hepatitis and with advanced rejection of the graft. She failed rapidly over the next 10 days despite medical therapy. His wife moribund in the intensive care unit, the husband arrived smelling of alcohol at the hospital to meet with the team members. He described his wife's nearly constant alcohol use and intermittent medication compliance since her surgery. At the family's request, one of the surgeons and the psychiatrist accompanied their two children with two child protection workers, together, to see their mother in the intensive care unit. She died 2 days later.

Perhaps the first clinical requirement that might have obviated this tragic outcome would have been an insistence on a face-to-face interview with the husband and the patient together. In an attempt to be kind to an impoverished family with young children, this was foregone in favor of a telephone conversation, a kindness never again repeated by the team. Dissembling can be done in person as well as by phone and, sadly, alcohol dependence is an easy condition to disguise or to minimize. No valid, non-historical indicators of alcohol dependence exist at present. From time to time research efforts have identified biological indicators that appear to be associated with heavy drinking; however, most of these indicators are very insensitive.

Table 3.8. *Reported experience with CDT as a marker for recent heavy alcohol use*

Study power	Sensitivity (%)	Specificity (%)	Positive predictive (%)
CDT levels			
Stibler *et al.* (1988a,b 1989))	83		
Behrens *et al.* (1988a)	79		
Behrens *et al.* (1988b)	81	91	89
Schellenberg *et al.* (1989)	76	90	
CDT/TST ratio			
Schellenberg *et al.* (1987)	82	88	
Schellenberg *et al.* (1989)	76	90	
Kwoh-Gain *et al.* (1990)	81	97	96

CDT: carbohydrate deficient transferrin; TST: total sum transferrin.

Recent studies have suggested the use of carbohydrate deficient transferrin (CDT) measurement, or the ratio of CDT to the total serum transferrin (TST) level, as a clinically valid indicator of heavy drinking having taken place within 2 weeks of the test (Stibler, 1991; Table 3.8). While controversy exists as to the best method of assessing this carrier protein, it appears to offer the best physical indication of recent heavy drinking that can be used in the follow-up care of liver graft recipients. The test appears to have limited usefulness in patients who are using alcohol in small to moderate quantities daily. This in turn may limits its helpfulness in recognizing 'socially drinking' liver transplantation patients. Other studies of non-cirrhotic alcoholics have suggested the use of liver enzyme changes over time as measures of drinking, an approach that seems to be obviated by liver transplant in this patient group.

Despite the likelihood that CDT or other markers will presumably become useful as indicators of an acute drinking episode, the concern that the patient is not telling the truth will still bother clinicians from time to time. For some clinicians it may become an insurmountable problem that may lead them to turn away alcohol dependent persons from consideration for transplant. While concerns of this nature are generally felt, members of our team and those of others with whom we communicate have been routinely surprised at the forthrightness with which most alcohol dependent patients will present their histories. This derives in part from an approach by the transplant team to the patient in which it is clearly stated that any and all conditions bearing on the transplant are likely to have serious implications for ultimate survival. As a result, it is in the patient's interest to be as honest as possible when discussing their alcohol use. The same approach can be communicated to the family of the patient. The statement itself is not a fiction because, as discussed elsewhere in this volume, alcoholic subjects require more extensive evaluation than non-alcoholics with regard to alcohol-related conditions such as cardiomyopathy. Recalling once again that the relationship between the drinker and the alcohol is an ambivalent one, there is much leeway from the point of view of survival that can allow the alcoholic to come to terms with the extent of his or her difficulty and the possibilities of improvement. We believe this approach is part of a unique circumstance of liver transplant provision and one which can be readily used to both the patient's and the team's advantage.

Change during the evaluation period

Drinking behavior is never a static phenomenon. The evaluation for transplant can of itself be a powerful agent in bringing the problem of uncontrolled drinking into focus for alcoholic candidates. Some patients who have ignored, minimized or failed to recognize an alcohol dependency beforehand, make use of the transplant crisis to control their drinking habit, as in the following case.

Case 3.4. This 45-year-old married mother of two children was admitted to hospital with liver failure. Biopsy showed alcoholic cirrhosis and the psychiatric history clearly showed alcohol dependence. Reviewing this information with her doctors, she commented that she had never regarded alcohol use as a problem and felt that she could stop whenever she wished. The doctors recommended alcohol rehabilitation which she refused. She was discharged home and given a follow-up appointment 3 months later. One week later she phoned her internist to say that she and her family had come to grips with her problem and that she wanted a treatment referral as soon as possible. She entered treatment the following week and did well. She received a liver graft 8 months later. She is alive, abstaining from alcohol and well 3 years later.

When cases of this kind occur, it is useful to provide either treatment or a referral for treatment as a way of helping patients make the changes required in their lives that are necessary to support long-term abstinence. We have noted cases in which resolution of the basic ambivalence toward drinking did not occur until after a transplant, as discussed in more detail below. In general, the opportunity for coming to grips with the presence of an alcohol dependency, for resolving the ambivalence toward the alcohol use and the behavior associated with it and for beginning the movement towards long-term abstinence, is usually a function of the physical health of the individual during the pre-transplant period and the time course dictated by the severity of their liver disease. For many, it is possible medically to stabilize the liver illness to make time available for a more lengthy evaluation and the possibility of change.

It is also sometimes the case that resumption of drinking occurs during the evaluation period.

Case 3.5. This 42-year-old alcoholic woman, who presented with mild encephalopathy, at first minimized her alcohol use but subsequently described it in detail after the psychiatrist contacted her husband to corroborate the history. She completed an extensive evaluation and was placed on the list for liver transplant with the strong recommendation that she attend treatment for her alcohol dependence after the surgery. Two months later the internist noted alcohol on her breath; her blood level was 20 mg/dl. Asked to return 1 week later, her blood alcohol level was 69 mg/dl. Presented with this information, she at first angrily refused to acknowledge her drinking. She was removed from the waiting list.

Most programs view this is as a very serious prognostic sign. When the evaluation has been completed, there is no doubt among the transplant team members as to the clarity of understanding of the problem of alcohol dependence both for the patient and the family members. When alcohol dependent candidates who have been accepted and placed on the list for transplant show evidence of resumed drinking, most programs will remove the patient from the list of those being considered. Having removed the person from the transplant list, possible patient care options may include a re-evaluation and follow-up assessment or a recommendation against the procedure. Some programs will elect to re-evaluate but will require a more stringent examination of the possibility of alcohol rehabilitation treatment before transplant can be recommended. Fortunately, our program has seen relatively few instances of this circumstance.

Results of selection

Over a 5-year period, from 1987 through the first part of 1992, we applied the above selection criteria to a series of transplant candidates, most of whom were alcohol dependent or abusive. Table 3.9 lists the frequencies with which the sample would have been denied a transplanted liver had any one of the prognostic factors served as the sole inclusion criteria. The actual rate of excluding alcoholic candidates from liver transplant for psychosocial reasons is approximately 16% or about one in six. Vaillant's prognostic factors were the most liberal and would have ruled out one in ten. One of every five patients did not recognize their alcoholism while nearly one in three presented unstable social

Table 3.9. *Prognostic factors of 233 alcohol abuse/dependence candidates*

Prognostic factor	*n*	%
Denial of alcohol dependence	43	18.5
Social stability score 2 or less	74	31.8
Vaillant's factors, 1 or none	23	9.9
Total index score <12	50	21.5
Actual rate of exclusion	37	15.9

Table 3.10. *Abuse/dependence comparisons of the prognosis*

	Abuse (n=35) *n* (%)	Dependence (n=198) *n* (%)
Vaillant's factors, 1 or none	1 (2.9)	16 (8.1)
Social stability score 2 or less	4 (11.4)	66 (33.3)

situations according to the Strauss–Bacon scale. The Total Index Score, a compilation of the first three factors, approximates a refusal rate of one in five. Two conclusions seem warranted. First, a majority of those referred are 'good prognosis' patients when considering factors that, to the best of our knowledge, support long-term abstinence. Second, the range among the various factors is too wide to justify using any one as a strict inclusion or exclusion criterion. While each of the factors, and indeed the Total Index Score, have useful contributions to make, inclusion or exclusion must entail a case-by-case assessment, discussion and decision by the transplant team.

The diagnostic dichotomy between abuse and dependence, suggesting that abuse is a more ameliorative diagnosis, derives some support from a comparison of the relative frequencies of the prognostic factors assessed among the same groups (Table 3.10). About 3% of the abuse group had only one or none of Vaillant's prognostic factors compared with nearly three times that proportion among the dependent group. The same proportion held true for patients with a Strauss–Bacon score of two or less. The actual frequencies among the abuse group are too small for tests of statistical significance but the trend warrants further study of what appears to be a useful clinical distinction.

The likelihood of ultimate selection for liver transplant can be seen as a triage process when considering the application of Vaillant's prognostic fac-

Table 3.11. *Vaillant's prognostic factors in 190 alcohol dependent patients listed for transplant*

No. of factors	*n*	Listed	%*n*
4	63	35	56
3	52	20	38
2	61	21	34
None or 1	14	2	14

tors. Table 3.11 shows the frequencies of the factors along with the number and frequency of patients accepted for liver transplant. The lowest acceptance rate mirrors the worst prognosis score. The acceptance rate more than doubles for those with two or three of Vaillant's factors and increases again for those appearing to have the best prognosis. The average acceptance rate for all groups is 41.1%. One recalls the origin of the triage process: the surgeon in the First World War facing massive numbers of casualties with limited resources allocating them where they will be most effective.

While it is tempting to view the numbers in Table 3.11 as bearing out the wisdom of the selection procedure, this ignores a circularity of reasoning that lives within them: acceptance for the procedure depends on the assessment of prognosis. The two are not arrived at independently. While scores were assigned for research purposes only and not presented in any clinical forum, the details of the prognostic outlook for each patient became part of the discussion of acceptance for liver transplant. The same circularity necessarily occurs in the discussion of psychiatric outcome (Chapter 6). The only way to solve this dilemma is to create two independent variables – acceptance for transplant and prognostic assessment. To do this hepatic transplants must be given randomly in a fashion that is blind to the prognostic assessment. It is at this point that scientific rigor outdistances ethical reserve. To randomize within the bounds of ethics, the physicians and surgeons must be equally poised between two comparably effective alternative treatment methods. As survival analysis data in this volume shows, there is no other equally effective treatment or lack of treatment. It the absence of the possibility of randomized assignment, we are best guided by the natural history of those patients who undergo the evaluation process and who are then assessed prospectively. Chapter 6 discusses the present state of knowledge of the postoperative course.

References

Arria, A. M., Tarter, R. E., Starzl, T. E. and Van, T. D. (1991). Improvement in cognitive functioning of alcoholics following orthotopic liver transplantation. *Alcoholism: Clinical and Experimental Research*, **15**, 956–62.

Behrens, U.J., Worner, T.M.,, Braly, L.F., Schaffner, F. and Lieber, C.S. (1988a). Carbohydrate-deficient transferrin, a marker for chronic alcohol consumption in different ethnic populations. *Alcoholism: Clnical and Experimental Research*, **12**, 427–32.

Behrens, U.J., Worner, T.M., Lieber, C.S. (1988b) Changes in carbohydrate-deficient transferrin levels after alcohol withdrawal. *Alcoholism: Clnical and Experimental Research*, **12**, 539–44.

Beresford, T. P., Schwartz, J., Wilson, D., Merion, M. and Lucey, M.R. (1992). The short-term psychological health of alcoholic and non-alcoholic liver transplant recipients. *Alcoholism: Clinical and Experimental Research*, **16**, 996–1000.

Beresford, T. P., Turcotte, J. G., Merion, R., Burtch, G., Blow, F. C., Campbell, D., Brower, K. J., Coffman, K. and Lucey, M. (1990). A rational approach to liver transplantation for the alcoholic patient. *Psychosomatics*, **31**, 241–54.

Bird, G. L., O'Grady, J. G., Harvey, F. A., Calne, R. Y. and Williams, R. (1990). Liver transplantation in patients with alcoholic cirrhosis: selection criteria and rates of survival and relapse. *British Medical Journal*, **301**, 15–7.

Folstein, M.F., Folstein, S.E. and McHugh, P.R. (1975). 'Mini-Mental State': a practical method for grading the cognitive state of patients for the clinician. *Journal of Psychiatric Research*, **12**, 189–98.

Frank, J. (1991). *Persuasion and Healing*, 3rd ed., rev. Baltimore, Johns Hopkins University Press.

Kwoh-Gain, I., Fletcher, L.M., Price, J., Powell, L.W. and Halliday, J.W. (1990). Desialylated transferrin and mitochondrial aspartate aminotransferase compared as laboratory markers of excessive alcohol consumption. *Clinical Chemistry*, **36**, 841–5.

Kumar, S., Stauber, R. E., Gavaler, J. S., Basista, M. H., Dindzans, V. J., Schade, R. R., Rabinovitz, M., Tarter, R. E., Gordon, R., Starzl, T. E. *et al.* (1990). Orthotopic liver transplantation for alcoholic liver disease. *Hepatology*, **11**, 159–64.

Lucey, M. R., Merion, R. M., Henley, K. S., Campbell, D. J., Turcotte, J. G., Nostrant, T. T., Blow, F. C. and Beresford, T. P. (1992). Selection for and outcome of liver transplantation in alcoholic liver disease. *Gastroenterology*, **102**, 1736–41.

Makela, K. and Room, R. (1985). Alcohol policy and the rights of the drunkard. *Alcoholism: Clinical and Experimental Research*, **9**, 2–5.

McCurry, K.R., Baliga, P., Merion, R.M., Ham, J.M., Lucey, M.R. Beresford, T.P., Turcotte, J.G. and Campbell, D.A. Jr (1992). Resource utilization and outcome of liver transplantation for alcoholic cirrhosis, a case-control study. *Archives of Surgery*, **127**, 772–6.

Mentha, G., Le Coultre, C., Huber, O., Meyer, P., Belli, D., Klopfenstein, C., Kowalski, M., Rohner, A. (1991) Orthotope Lebertransplantation—Indikationen und Resultate. *Schweiz Rundsch Med Prax*, **80**, 1380–7.

Mirza, D.F., Goetzinger, P., Fuegger, R., Wamser, P., Steininger, R. and Muehlbacher, F. (1991). Orthotopic liver transplantation in the management of end stage liver disease: the University of Vienna experience. *Indian Journal of Gastroenterology*, **10**, 92–5.

Polich, J. M., Armor, D.J. and Braker, H.B. (1981). *The Course Of Alcoholism: Four Years After Treatment*. New York, Wiley.

Schellenberg, F., Benard, J.Y., Le Goff, A.M., Bourdin, C. and Weill, J. (1989). Evaluation of carbohydrate-deficient transferrin compared with Tf index and other markers of alcohol abuse. *Alcoholism: Clinical and Experimental Research*, **10**, 61–4.

Schellenberg, F. and Weill, J. (1987). Serum desialotransferrin in the detection of alcohol abuse. Definition of a Tf index. *Drug and Alcohol Dependence*, **19**, 181–91.

Schuckit, M.A. (1991). *Drug and Alcohol Abuse. A Clinical Guide to Diagnosis and Treatment*, 3rd edn. New York, Plenum Press.

Skinner, H.A., Holt, S. and Israel, Y. (1981). Early identification of alcohol abuse. 1. Critical issues and psychosocial indicators for a composite index. *Canadian Medical Assocociation Journal*, **124**, 1141–52.

Starzl, T. E., Van, T. D., Tzakis, A. G., Iwatsuki, S., Todo, S., Marsh, J. W., Koneru, B., Staschak, S., Stieber, A. and Gordon, R. D. (1988). Orthotopic liver transplantation for alcoholic cirrhosis. *Journal of the American Medical Association*, **260**, 2542–4.

Smith, E.M. and Cloninger, C.R, (1985). A prospective twelve-year follow-up of alcoholic women: a prognostic scale for long-term outcome. *NIDA Research Monograph*, **55**, 245–51.

Stibler, H. (1991). Carbohydrate-deficient transferrin in serum: a new marker of potentially harmful alcohol consumption reviewed. *Clinical Chemistry*, **37**, 2029–37.

Stibler, H. and Borg, S. (1986). Carbohydrate composition of serum transferrin in alcoholic patients. *Alcoholism: Clinical and Experimental Research*, **10**, 61–4.

Stibler, H., Borg, S. and Beckman, G. (1988a). Transferrin phenotype and level of carbohydrate-deficient transferrin in healthy individuals. *Alcoholism: Clinical and Experimental Research*, **12**, 450–3.

Stibler, H., Dahlgren, L. and Borg, S. (1988b) Carbohydrate-deficient transferrin (CDT) in serum in women with early alcohol addiction. *Alcohol*, **5**, 393–8.

Strauss, R. and Bacon S.D. (1951). Alcoholism and social stability. *Quarterly Journal of the Study of Alcohol*, **12**, 231–60.

Trzepacz, P. T., Brenner, R. and Van Thiel, D. (1989). A psychiatric study of 247 liver transplantation candidates. *Psychosomatics*, **30**, 147–53.

Vaillant, G. (1983). *The Natural History Of Alcoholism* . Cambridge, MA, Harvard University Press.

Vaillant, G. E. (1988). What can long-term follow-up teach us about relapse and prevention of relapse in addiction? *British Journal of Addiction*, **83**, 1147–57.

Vaillant, G.E., Clark, W., Cyrus, C., Kopp, J., Wustin, V.W., Milotsky, E.S., and Mogielnicki, N.P. (1983). Prospective study of alcoholism treatment: eight year follow-up. *American Journal of Medicine*, **75**, 455–63.

CHAPTER FOUR

MEDICAL ASSESSMENT OF ALCOHOLIC CANDIDATES FOR LIVER TRANSPLANTATION

MICHAEL R. LUCEY

Introduction

The aims of medical evaluation for liver transplantation of patients with putative alcoholic liver disease are: (1) to establish the diagnosis of alcoholic liver disease, (2) to determine whether there are extrahepatic manifestations of alcohol-related end-organ damage, or indeed any significant medical conditions, which would impair recovery from liver transplantation, and (3) to estimate prognosis, with maximal medical and surgical therapy other than liver transplantation. Based on these judgments, the transplant physician can form an opinion on the patient's need for liver transplant and also the likelihood for a successful outcome. Finally, the members of the evaluation team should inform the patient of the risks and benefits of transplantation so that, should it be offered, the patient can make an informed decision. Encephalopathy may confound this process of education in some patients. I have specifically omitted the consideration of psychosocial suitability because it is the subject of a separate chapter. In reality, careful assessment of the psychosocial background of alcoholic patients is undertaken contemporaneously with medical assessment.

Defining alcoholic liver disease

Three inter-related conditions are usually included under this rubric - alcoholic fatty liver, acute alcoholic hepatitis and alcoholic cirrhosis. All three may coexist. The mechanisms which are thought to underlie the etiology of alcoholic liver disease will not be reviewed here (see Zakim *et al.*, 1990). It is worth considering the definition of alcoholic liver disease because it is a diagnosis which of itself may impact on the outcome of the evaluation. For example, the transplant evaluation team may be reluctant to accept for transplantation a patient with the diagnosis of alcoholic cirrhosis but find the same patient acceptable when the diagnosis is given as cryptogenic cirrhosis. Indeed, it is clear that house officers and students often have a negative attitude towards patients with alcoholism and it is reasonable to presume that this bias may also apply to more senior doctors and nurses (Geller *et al.*, 1989).

Unfortunately the grounds for making the diagnosis of alcoholic liver disease can be nebulous. Most commonly, the alcoholic patient referred for transplant evaluation will provide an unequivocal history of alcoholism, usually in a clinical setting of acute alcoholic hepatitis or cirrhosis, and there will be no doubt that the liver injury was caused by alcohol. In other circumstances, however, alcoholism and alcoholic liver disease need not be synonymous. Particular examples of this dichotomy are: (1) patients who have alcoholism without alcoholic liver disease, which is estimated to account for up to 90% of alcoholics, (2) alcoholic liver disease without alcoholism, i.e. characteristic features of alcoholic liver disease plus a history of heavy drinking which fails to meet the diagnostic criteria for alcoholism (see Chapter 2 for a

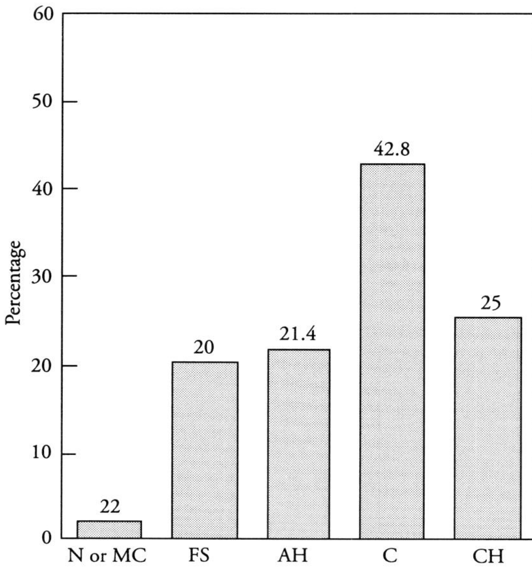

Figure 4.1. Prevalence of anti-HCV antibodies in alcoholic patients according to the degree of damage on liver biopsy. N or MC: normal or minimal changes; FS: fibrosteatosis; AH: alcoholic hepatitis; C: cirrhosis; CH: chronic hepatitis. p <0.001. Reproduced from Pares *et al.* (1990) with permission.

full discussion of this), and (3) liver conditions which mimic alcoholic liver disease without a history of alcohol abuse or even alcohol consumption (Powell *et al.*, 1990).

A further complexity to the definitions of alcoholic liver disease is that alcoholics are at risk for the development of non-alcoholic liver disease. For example, evidence from Spain suggests that up to 40% of patients with alcoholic cirrhosis are infected with Hepatitis C virus (Pares *et al.*, 1990) (Figure 4.1). Among the implications of this observation are first, that in some cases at least, alcoholic cirrhosis may be caused by environmental factors that are beyond the control of the patient. Second, it indicates that a careful search for other liver diseases is necessary in patients with alcoholic cirrhosis. Finally, the risk of recurrence of non-alcoholic liver disease in the alcoholic recipient may modify selection, pretransplant management or post-transplant management.

Alternatively, alcoholic liver disease may be defined by estimating the total alcohol dose consumed. In this case, liver disease is presumed to have been caused by alcohol when it has occurred in someone whose consumption has exceeded a predetermined threshold. This definition does not circumvent the problems posed by other environmental factors such as Hepatitis C virus (HCV). Nonetheless, much of the epidemiologic evidence suggests that there is a link between the amount of alcohol consumed and the frequency of alcohol-induced damage (Powell and Klatskin, 1968; Alexander *et al.*, 1971). The association between total dose of alcohol consumed and alcoholic liver injury is not substantiated, however, in all prospective studies. Sorenson *et al.* (1984) found that the progression to alcoholic cirrhosis in male alcoholics was independent of the total alcohol dose above a threshold of 50 g alcohol a day for 1 year. Moreover, women appear to develop alcohol-induced liver injury at lower daily intakes than men (Loft *et al.*, 1987), which Lieber and coworkers have attributed to differences in gastric alcohol dehydrogenase activity between men and women (Frezza *et al.*, 1990). Finally, self-reported alcohol history by alcoholics is notoriously inaccurate (Orrego *et al.*, 1979). For these reasons it is unsatisfactory to rely on reported consumption as the sole diagnostic criterion on which to diagnose alcoholic liver disease.

Even liver biopsy, the cornerstone of diagnosis of alcoholic liver disease, is not an absolute arbiter. As mentioned above, alcoholic liver disease may be subcategorized into acute alcoholic hepatitis, alcoholic fatty liver and alcoholic cirrhosis. In practice, these categories often overlap in the same biopsy. A second problem is that the characteristic features of alcoholic liver disease are not exclusive to alcohol-induced damage. Typical appearances of alcoholic liver disease may be found in postjejunoileal bypass patients who develop liver injury, in some drug reactions (amiodarone and perhexaline are examples of drugs which may cause an alcoholic-like lesion) and in some patients for whom the cause in unclear but who give no history of alcohol use. The latter entity has been given the acronym NASH (non-alcoholic steatohepatitis). Female sex, obesity and diabetes mellitus are predisposing factors (Diehl *et al.*, 1988; Powell *et al.*, 1990). The biopsy features of NASH include macrovesicular fat deposition, Mallory's hyaline and a lobular inflammatory infiltrate. Although progression to cirrhosis is rare, some fibrosis is often present. Thus a liver biopsy may reveal characteristic features of alcoholic liver injury but it cannot establish beyond all doubt that alcohol is the cause of that injury.

The distinction between alcoholic and non-alcoholic injury is also an important reason to perform a liver biopsy. For example, distinguishing alcoholic liver disease with secondary hemosiderosis from primary hereditary hemochromatosis requires a liver biopsy and the iron content quantified (Bassett *et al.*, 1986). The calculation of the 'hepatic iron index' is a useful method of discriminating between hereditary hemochromatosis and secondary

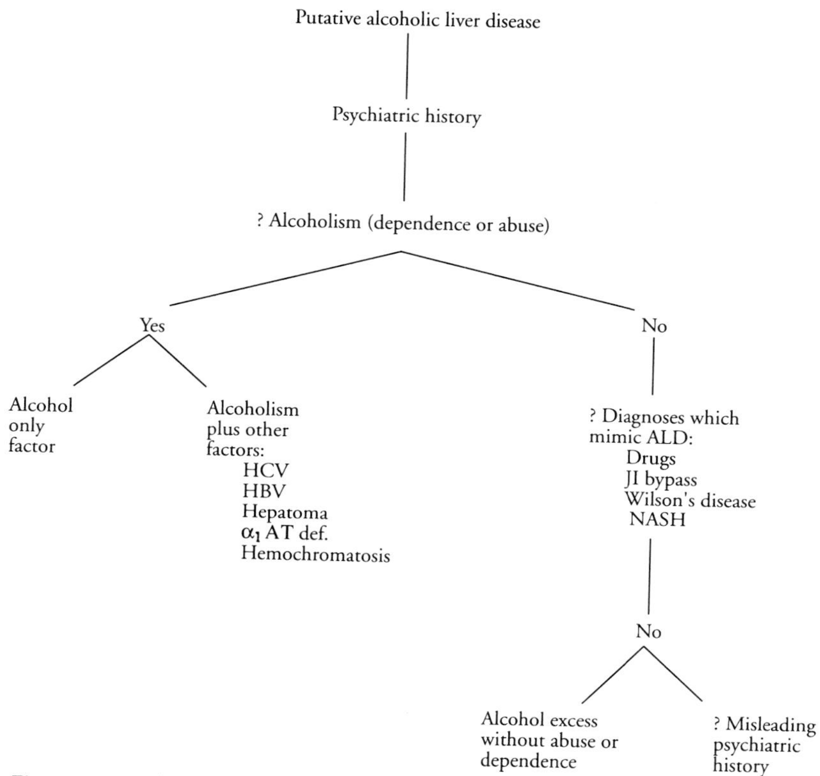

Figure 4.2. An algorhithm to determine if alcohol is a cause of liver damage in a person with a putative diagnosis of alcoholic liver disease. α_1 AT def.: alpha$_1$ antitrypsin deficiency; ALD: alcoholic liver disease; JI: jejunoileal.

hemosiderosis due to alcohol. Liver biopsy may also assist when estimating the prognosis of alcoholic liver disease. Continued alcohol intake by persons with a combination of steatosis and acute alcoholic hepatitis is associated with an 80% chance of developing cirrhosis (Sorenson *et al.*, 1984).

In our programme, we have defined alcoholism as alcohol dependence or abuse according to DSM-III-R (see Chapters 2 and 3). Alcoholic liver disease is defined as acute or chronic liver disease in alcohol dependent or abusive patients in whom no other more likely cause of liver injury has been discovered. Other causes of liver injury are searched for in every patient (e.g. viral hepatitis, hemochromatosis, etc). Patients with clinical features of alcoholic liver disease (characteristic liver biopsy, a ratio of aspartate aminotransferase

(AST) to alanine aminotransferase (ALT) which exceeds two) who deny dependence or abuse are kept under review. Examples such as amiodarone toxicity or jejunoileal bypass hepatopathy are rare and not likely to be confused with alcoholism. In most cases, where doubt about the diagnosis of alcoholic liver disease arises, it is because of doubt about the truthfulness of the psychiatric history (see Chapter 2). New information may come to light while evaluating these patients which contradicts the previous history (for example when a patient who was previously denying alcohol use presents to clinic with a measurable blood alcohol level or when a history of excessive drinking by the patient undergoing evaluation is received from a family member) necessitating a new diagnostic formulation; the outcome of liver transplant evaluation may change accordingly. Occasionally, despite liver biopsy and other evidence to suggest possible alcoholic injury, the patient will consistently deny alcohol use. When this occurs in a clinical setting typical of NASH, a working diagnosis of NASH will be made (see vignette case 2.1, p. 13). An algorhythm to outline this plan is shown in Figure 4.2.

Extra hepatic complications of alcoholism

Cardiomyopathy

Cardiomyopathy is reported to be common in actively drinking alcoholics. For example, Urbano-Marquez *et al.* (1989) found an ejection fraction of less than 55% in one-third of 50 actively drinking alcoholic men whereas none of the 20 control males had an ejection fraction of less than 55%. Similar prospective data on the incidence of alcoholic cardiomyopathy in consecutive alcoholic patients undergoing liver transplantation are not available. In our own center, all alcoholic patients considered for liver transplantation undergo cardiologic assessment unless they are excluded for other reasons. In a retrospective review of 101 adult patients who underwent cardiac evaluation between 1988 and 1990, 43 were alcoholic according to DSM-III-R criteria. Abnormalities on electrocardiography and/or multiple equilibrium-gated radionuclide angiography (MUGA) were present in 36 (84%) of the alcoholic and in 39 (64%) of the non-alcoholic candidates. The most common abnormalities were ischemic changes or rhythm/conduction abnormalities observed in electrocardiographs; they were equally distributed in both groups. Significant abnormalities on echocardiography were uncommon in both alcoholic and non-alcoholic patients. For example, abnormalities of the chambers (enlargement, hypertrophy or poor wall motion) were observed in seven alcoholics (16%) and in eight non-alcoholics (14%). One alcoholic patient only was not selected for transplantation on cardiac grounds and this was because of accompanying ischemic heart disease. The survival of patients post-transplant seemed to be unaffected by the presence or absence of cardiac abnormalities in the pretransplant evaluation. However, this retrospective analysis may not be sufficiently robust to determine whether specific subtle cardiologic abnormalities portend intraoperative or postoperative complications.

A further likely reason for the rarity of alcoholic cardiomyopathy in our series may be the influence of alcohol withdrawal on cardiac muscle function in alcoholics. A specific period of abstinence has not been required for an alcoholic patient to be considered for evaluation in our program but most alcoholic patients referred to us who undergo a full cardiac evaluation have stopped drinking for over 6 months. This period of abstinence may allow recovery of the cardiac muscle.

Finally, we may have observed a lower than expected incidence of alcoholic cardiomyopathy because of biases in selection of alcoholic patients who are referred by primary and secondary care physicians to a transplant center. This process may select alcoholics with a lower incidence of alcoholic cardiomyopathy. In summary, although there is a paucity of data on the cardiomyopathy among alcoholics undergoing evaluation for liver transplantation, our impression is that alcoholic cardiomyopathy has proven to be a less significant problem than anticipated. There is a clear need for a prospective study of cardiac function in alcoholic and non-alcoholic patients about to undergo liver transplantation and, until this is done, we to recommend electrocardiography and echocardiography in all alcoholic persons undergoing evaluation for liver transplantation.

Myopathy

Alcoholic myopathy is common in actively drinking alcoholics and may be related to total dose of ethanol consumed (Urbano-Marquez *et al.,* 1989). Nonetheless, it is not commonly a factor which determines suitability.

Pancreatitis

Alcoholic pancreatitis, although an important cause of morbidity among alcoholics, is not a clinical feature which directly impacts on the decision to offer or withhold transplantation.

Osteopenia

The incidence of osteopenia and the frequency of skeletal bone fractures are increased in persons with alcoholic liver disease when compared with non-alcoholic controls (Bonkovsky *et al.*, 1990; Diamond *et al.*, 1990). The reasons for these phenomena are multiple including defective vitamin D metabolism, impaired nutritional status and defective osteoblast function (Compston, 1986). Diamond and coworkers assessed the dynamics of bone formation and absorption in actively drinking alcoholics and compared them with two control groups, inactive alcoholics and non-drinkers. Active drinkers had significantly less osteoblastic activity than abstainers as assessed by dynamic bone histomorphometry (Diamond *et al.*, 1989). These data suggest that ethanol or its metabolites may be responsible for impaired osteoblastic activity which may contribute to the osteopenia observed in alcoholic cirrhotics. As discussed in Chapter 6, the presence of osteopenia before operation is a cause of concern because this state is likely to deteriorate in the postoperative recovery period when high dose glucocorticoids are administered (Porayko *et al.*, 1991). The presence of significant bone disease may occasionally be a factor in refusal to select a candidate for liver transplantation.

Common medical problems in alcoholics

Infection

Bacterial infection

Sepsis is a contraindication to transplantation other than rare cases in which infection is confined to the biliary tract. Careful evaluation for septic foci (spontaneous bacterial peritonitis, hepatic abscess, infectious endocarditis) may be an important part of the transplant evaluation. All alcoholic candidates have a PPD (purified protein derivative) placed because tuberculosis is common among alcoholics.

Viral and other infections

Many alcoholic persons with end-stage liver disease have concomitant viral hepatitis which may be caused by a history of illicit drug use. It is not uncommon to find serum markers for hepatitis C, B and/or D (HCV, HBV, HDV) in alcoholic patients undergoing transplant evaluation. Serum human immunodeficiency virus (HIV) antibody and antibodies to CMV, Epstein-Barr virus (EBV), Herpes simplex virus (HSV), varicella and toxoplasma are estimated routinely.

The impact of a positive result of any of these tests differs according to the infection in question. Indeed it is likely that any current protocol will be modified in the future as more information about specific pathogens is gained and there are advances in therapeutics and immunosuppression. For example, it is our policy at present, not to offer liver transplants to HIV antibody positive persons, even though moderate short term success has been reported when HIV-infected persons have been given liver transplants either knowingly or inadvertently (Tzakis *et al.*, 1990). In contrast, we have not withheld liver transplantation from patients with HBV infection despite a very frequent incidence of HBV infection in the graft (Davis *et al.*, 1991). In our own series of 17 grafts in 15 serum HBsAg positive subjects, which included 5 alcoholic recipients, HBV infection occurred in 13 grafts (Lucey *et al.*, 1992b). Active viral replication as shown by either the presence of HBeAg or HBV DNA in serum or HBcAg in liver, is associated with frequent graft infection, whereas a fulminant presentation or concomitant HDV infection appears to reduce the chances of significant graft infection or injury. Recently, Samuel *et al.* have reported in a non-controlled clinical study that long term administration of high doses of HBIg to recipients at risk of HBV infection reduced the incidence of graft infection (Samuel *et al.*, 1991). It is likely that future clinical studies will define what factors predict the risk of graft infection by HBV and of progressive liver injury in grafts which have become so infected.

The significance of HCV antibodies in alcoholics with liver disease has been the cause of controversy. With the advent of second generation antibody tests and confirmation of active infection by polymerase chain reaction (PCR)-amplification of HCV RNA, it is has become clear that many alcoholics are infected with HCV (Pares *et al.*, 1990). Furthermore, there is a correlation between the coincidence of HCV infection and the severity of liver injury. For example, in the study of Pares *et al.* from Spain, HCV antibodies were present in 2.2% of alcoholics with normal liver histology, approximately 20% of those with fibrosteatosis or alcoholic hepatitis but in 42.6% of those with cirrhosis (Figure 4.1). Nishiguchi *et al.* (1991) workers have reported very similar results from Japan. They found HCV antibodies in 1 of 10 alcoholic patients with fibrosteatosis, 2 of 20 with acute alcoholic hepatitis, 15 of 19 with chronic hepatitis and 18 of 31 with cirrhosis and confirmed that these results represented active infection by testing the same sera for HCV RNA using nested PCR. Thus, the incidence of HCV antibodies in alcoholic cirrhotics was in both studies remarkably similar at (43% and 61%, respectively) and the second study confirmed that this was indicative of active infection and not a false positive result.

Just as HBV and HDV can recur after transplantation, HCV frequently recurs in the grafted liver, and given their high incidence of HCV, alcoholic cirrhotics are particularly at risk. Martin *et al.* (1991) described six liver transplant recipients who were HCV antibody-positive before operation in four of whom the pretransplant diagnosis was alcoholic liver disease. All six remained HCV antibody-positive post-transplant. One recipient had severe post-transplant hepatitis leading to loss of the graft and ultimately death and two recipients had mild or intermittent hepatic features. Other studies have also shown that chronic hepatitis is common in hepatitis C-infected liver grafts but that it usually takes a more indolent course than HBV infection (Feray *et al.*, 1992; Wright *et al.*, 1992b). It is our practice, therefore, to measure serum HCV antibodies in all alcoholic candidates. While a positive result indicates an increased risk of post-transplant hepatitis, it is not a sufficient reason to refuse transplantation. Although HCV may be suppressed in some immunocompetent patients by administration of interferon alpha (Shindo *et al.*, 1991), data for pre- or post-transplant use of interferon alpha in HCV antibody-positive candidates are not encouraging (Wright *et al.*, 1992a).

The principal risk factor for the development of post-transplant cytomegalovirus (CMV) infection of the liver is the presence of CMV antibody in the donor (Gorensek *et al.*, 1990). The risk of developing significant CMV infection when a recipient (alcoholic or not) receives a liver from a CMV antibody-positive donor may be ameliorated by prophylaxis using intravenous immune globulin for 6 weeks and acyclovir for up to 6 months (Stratta *et al.*, 1991). The remaining pretransplant antibody titres (EBV, HSV, varicella, toxoplasmosis) serve as a useful bench mark when investigating the cause of hepatitis in the post-transplant period.

Hepatoma

Alcoholic cirrhotics are at increased risk for the development of hepatoma. The reasons for this may in part be related to: (1) clandestine HBV infection (Brechot *et al.*, 1982) or more probably to the frequency of HCV infection in alcoholic cirrhotics because HCV may itself be a risk factor for hepatoma (Colombo *et al.*, 1991). Alcohol cirrhotic persons undergoing evaluation for liver transplantation, especially those in whom there has been an acute clinical deterioration, must be carefully screened for hepatoma. The coexistence of HBV or HCV infection, or hemachromatosis should increase the index of suspicion. Serum alpha-fetoprotein and either real time ultrasonography or contrast-enhanced CT of the abdomen is a reasonable starting point when screening for hepatoma. Standard angiography probably offers little additional benefit unless a lesion has already been recognized and the presence of vessel encasement is being determined. The role of more sophisticated imaging modalities, such as magnetic resonance imagin (MRI) or computerized tomography (CT) scan following selective angiographic injection of lipiodol, have yet to be defined but may be useful in selected cases. Cytological analysis of ascites from cirrhotics at risk of developing hepatoma is appropriate.

Once a lesion (or lesions) has been identified in the liver, the key questions are: (1) is it malignant, (2) is it unilocular or multilocular in the liver, (3) has it spread outside the liver, and (4) is it encapsulated. Tumors that have spread beyond the liver cannot be treated by liver transplantation. Controversies remain regarding the value of attempting transplantation in tumors confined to the liver. Before that question can be addressed for an individual patients, a decision has to be made on whether to seek a tissue diagnosis, especially as there is a risk of dissemmation of malignant tumors by the biopsy needle. It can be argued that it would be wise to forego a biopsy whenever transplantation would be undertaken irrespective of the outcome of the biopsy. Nonetheless, we frequently choose to confirm by aspiration or biopsy the nature of a suspicious lesion.

A more difficult circumstance is that in which the patient with well-compensated cirrhosis is found to have a suspicious lesion on ultrasound or CT scan but whose liver disease *per se* does not require transplantation. There is no consensus in the literature on the proper approach to investigation or, for that matter, treatment in this group of patients. Franco *et al.* (1990) reported a 60% 3-year survival rate among Child's class A cirrhotics undergoing primary resection of their tumor. A contrary view is taken by Van Thiel *et al.* (1991) who argue that imaging methods underestimate the frequency of vascular invasion and that liver transplant is the best mode of treatment for cirrhotic patients with small hepatomas confined to the liver (Belli *et al.*, 1989). Indeed, the Pittsburgh group argue against selection for transplantation of patients with large liver tumors but agree with selection of those patients with small tumours in whom there is hope for cure (Van Thiel *et al.*, 1991). Table 4.1 shows those features which indicate a good or poor prognosis after liver transplantation for patients with a hepatoma. (Van Thiel *et al.*, 1991)

There are no controlled data comparing liver transplantation with other forms of treatment for hepatoma. The series of patients with hepatoma treated by liver transplant often include patients in whom the presence of hepatoma was unknown before surgery. These patients with small unknown primaries are probably not comparable to patients who receive treatment for a defined

Table 4.1. *Prognostic factors for hepatoma treated by liver transplantation*

Prognostic factor
Good
Incidental finding during evaluation or in resected specimen
Lesion less than 5 cm in diameter
Single lesion
Presence of a capsule
Poor
Symptoms of cancer
Vascular invasion
Multiple lesions

Source: After Van Thiel *et al.* (1991).

hepatoma. Furthermore some authors subclassify hepatomas as incidental or non-incidental (Van Thiel *et al.*, 1991). By incidental is meant all previously unknown tumours discovered at laparotomy plus, in some studies, asymptomatic small tumours identified before operation. This confusing nomenclature makes comparison of outcome after treatment difficult both between series of patients with hepatomas treated by liver transplantation at different centers and also between transplantation and other modes of therapy (Di Bisceglie, 1991).

However, it is fair to say that liver transplantation is not contraindicated in all alcoholic cirrhotic persons in whom preoperative investigation reveals a small hepatoma, usually defined as less than 3 cms in diameter. Whether such patients would be better treated by primary resection or the other modalities mentioned above has not been tested in any comparative study. It is unlikely that any treatment in Child C patients such as chemoembolization, primary resection or directed chemotherapy, which does not correct the underlying liver disease, will have any long-term success. Unfortunately, when patients with known hepatomas undergo liver transplantation, tumor involvement within the allograft occurs frequently. Patients with cirrhosis and primary hepatic malignancy have a significantly reduced 2-year survival (O'Grady *et al.*, 1988; Ismail *et al.*, 1990; Olthoff *et al.*, 1990) (Figure 4.3). Thus, the role for transplantation in alcoholics with hepatoma remains uncertain. Indeed, most of these patients will not be selected for transplantation. In our series of 99 alcoholic cirrhotics assessed for transplantation from 1985 to 1989, two patients with an unknown (i.e. incidental) hepatoma were selected whereas five patients in whom hepatoma was discovered during evaluation were not chosen for transplantation (Lucey *et al.*, 1992a).

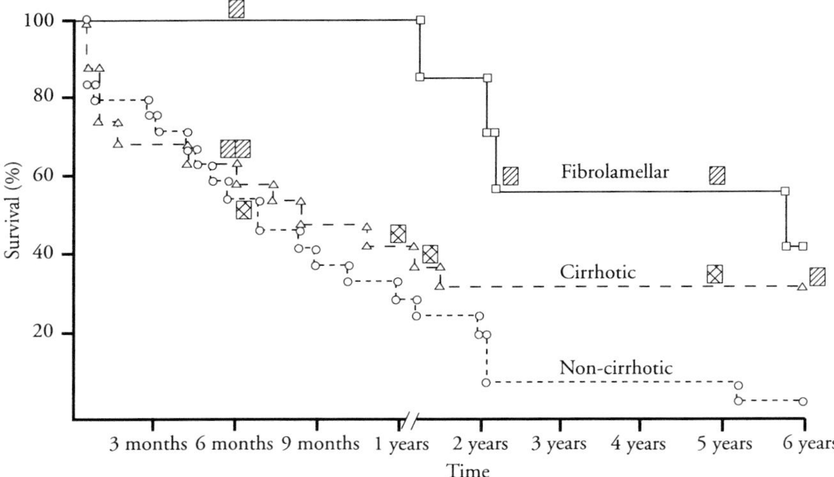

Figure 4.3. Kaplan–Meier survival curves for patients with hepatocellular carcinoma arising in cirrhotic or non-cirrhotic livers who subsequently underwent liver transplantation. (▨) Alive with no tumor recurrence. (⊠) Alive with tumor recurrence. Adapted from O'Grady *et al.* (1988) with permission.

Encephalopathy

When our transplant program began in 1985, chronic irreversible cerebral impairment was considered a contraindication to transplantation. Since then it has become clear that it is often impossible to distinguish fixed cerebral defects from chronic encephalopathy which will improve with restoration of hepatic function. Clinical and functional cerebral abnormalities are common in alcoholic cirrhosis (Charness, *et al.*, 1989; O'Carroll *et al.*, 1991). Improvement in encephalopathy after liver transplantation has been observed for alcoholics and non-alcoholics alike (Tarter *et al.*, 1990; Arria *et al.*, 1991). Indeed, even in a case of severe hepatocerebellar degeneration documented on CT scanning occurring 23 years after portosystemic shunting for non-alcoholic liver disease, liver transplantation significantly improved intellectual function and chronic neurologic signs (Powell *et al.*, 1990). Encephalopathy further confounds evaluation because it hinders estimation of insight into alcoholism and prognosis for future abstinence.

There is no consensus regarding the best method of evaluation of chronic encephalopaths for liver transplant. CT scanning is often used to identify focal cerebral injury. Single photon emission computerized tomography (SPECT),

MRI and position emission tomograpy (PET) scanning hold potential for improving the recognition of irreversible CNS lesions. Given the recorded response of encephalopathy to restoration of hepatic function, caution is necessary before a CNS lesion is considered permanent.

Prognosis from alcoholic liver disease

An important function of transplant evaluation is the estimation of prognosis as this judgment has considerable bearing on whether the evaluation team considers liver transplantation a suitable therapy for an individual patient. It is axiomatic that nobody wishes to transplant patients with many years potential survival without transplantation. In such cases transplantation poses a greater risk than conservative management. The estimated prognosis also influences timing of transplantation. Chosing the right time to place a patient on the waiting list is made more difficult by the paucity of donor organs and the unpredictable waiting period for each patient.

As I have described above, part of the evaluation process consists of searching for significant secondary diagnoses, such as viral hepatitis or hepatoma, which themselves may influence the overall prognosis. The impact of such phenomena on prognostic assessment will not be reiterated here.

Effect of continued alcohol use

Unfortunately, for most forms of acute or chronic liver disease, estimating prognosis is a very unexact art. Alcoholic liver disease is no exception. One confounding factor in almost all studies of prognosis in alcoholic liver disease is the difficulty in quantifying continued alcohol use. It might appear self-evident that continued drinking by alcoholics with liver disease will inevitably lead to further liver damage. The evidence to support this contention, however, has many flaws. Most studies that have addressed the effect of alcohol use on the survival of patients with alcoholic liver disease have relied on the patient's reported drinking habits to estimate abstinence or recidivism. Orrego *et al.* (1979) have shown that self-reporting by alcoholic cirrhotic patients underestimates true drinking. They showed, using daily urine samples, that among alcoholic cirrhotics who reported continued drinking, positive urines were common whereas those who claimed total abstinence also had some positive urines albeit less frequently. These data suggest that patient-reported history stratifies alcoholics into lesser and greater alcohol consumption cohorts rather than abstinent and actively drinking cohorts. The studies of Powell and

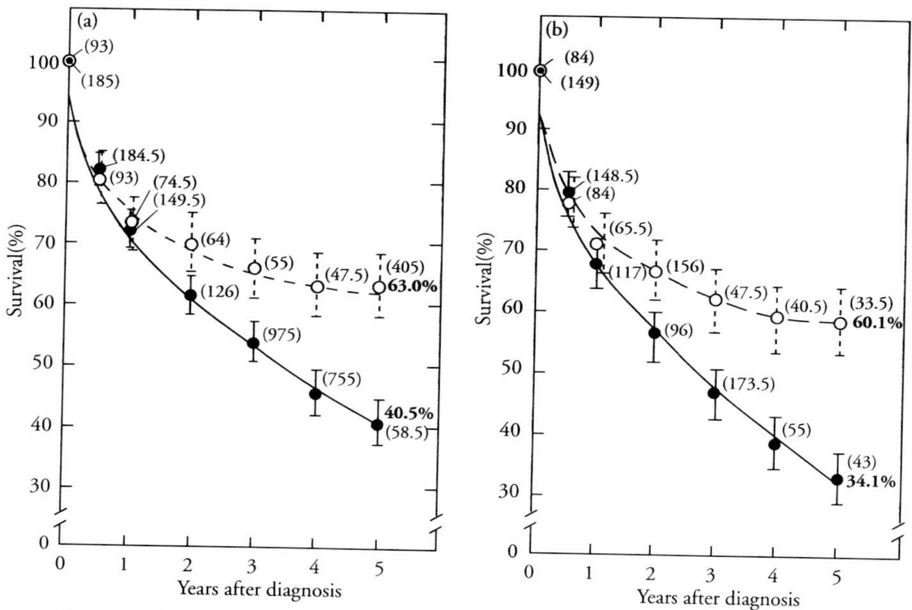

Figure 4.4. Survival after diagnosis of alcoholic cirrhosis in 278 patients (a) and in 233 patients from the onset of decompensation (b), stratified according to the patients' reported combined alcohol use or abstinence. (○- - -○) Stopped. (●——●) Continued. Reproduced from Powell and Klatskin (1968) with permission.

Klatskin which purported to show longer survival in abstinent alcoholic subjects when compared with alcoholics who continued to drink (63% vs 40.5% at 8 years) may have compared degrees of alcohol use rather than absolute use or non-use (Powell and Klatskin, 1968) (Figure 4.4). Indeed, subsequent studies using a similar self-report methodology have failed to demonstrate the benefit of (self-reported) abstinence (Soterakis *et al.*, 1973, Gines *et al.*, 1987). The retrospective nature of these studies, plus the uncertainties about how much alcohol was being consumed, make it impossible to reconcile the conflicting data. It should not be presumed that absolute abstinence is necessary for recovery or stabilization of liver injury. Reinterpreting Powell and Klatskin's observations as distinguishing between more heavy and less heavy alcohol use, raises the interesting possibility that there may be a threshold of alcohol consumption below which liver injury is minimized.

Support for the notion that factors other than dose of alcohol consumed mediate the onset of cirrhosis can be drawn from the prospective study of

Sorenson *et al.* (1984) in which persons with a daily alcohol consumption of greater than 50 g for 1 year and in whom liver biopsy did not show cirrhosis were followed for a median of 14 years. The authors showed that the degree of injury seen on biopsy rather than the reported duration of alcohol use or dose of alcohol consumed up to the time of entry into the study predicted the development of cirrhosis. The study is flawed, however, by lacking a measure of continued alcohol use in the observation period.

A further confounding factor has been the tendency to combine all forms of alcohol-related liver injury together when studying the effects of alcohol. This may mask differences of response to further alcohol exposure by subtypes of alcoholic injury. For example, Chedid *et al.* (1991) found among a cohort of 281 alcoholic men that continued alcohol use was a poor prognostic factor in patients with acute alcoholic hepatitis only. In those patients with either cirrhosis alone or acute alcoholic hepatitis plus cirrhosis, prognosis was independent of continued alcohol use.

Two studies, in which the confounding factors of severity of liver injury at study entry and accuracy of drinking history are recognized, deserve description. In the first, Alexander *et al.* (1971) described 157 patients with a clinical diagnosis of acute alcoholic hepatitis and separated them into 59 who stopped *or reduced* drinking and 98 who continued to drink as much as before. Estimated 5-year survival was 80% in the reduced drinking group compared with 60% in the continued drinking group (see Figure 4.5). Thus it seems likely that continued *heavy* alcohol intake is harmful to patients with acute alcoholic hepatitis. In the second study, Borowsky *et al.* (1981) surveyed 37 alcoholics with end-stage liver disease (all had ascites) after they had completed a program of detoxification. The alcoholics were stratified as continued heavy alcohol intake, moderate alcohol intake and abstinence and it was found that whereas continued heavy alcohol use was associated with increased mortality, abstainers and moderate users did not show excess mortality.

In summary, the data reviewed support the following conclusions. It is likely that continued heavy alcohol use is harmful to persons with alcoholic liver disease. This is particularly so for persons with acute alcoholic hepatitis and/or decompensated liver function. It is less certain that moderate alcohol use is harmful to persons with prior alcohol-related liver damage. The salutary effects on alcoholic liver disease of abstinence from alcohol compared with moderate use have not been demonstrated conclusively. This may be because of the difficulty of establishing a study cohort of alcoholics that does, in fact, abstain. It seems reasonable, therefore, to advocate abstinence from alcohol to all patients with alcoholic liver disease, pending better data,

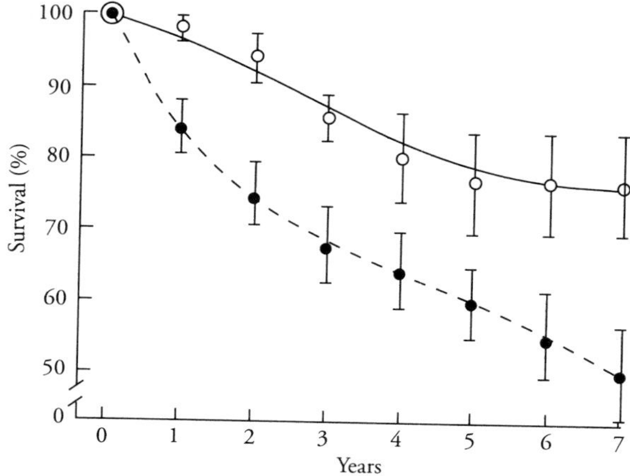

Figure 4.5. Survival in 59 patients with biopsy-documented acute alcoholic hepatitis stratified according to continued heavy drinking (- - -) or reduced intake/abstinence (—). Reproduced from Alexander *et al.* (1971) with permission.

because this course is the potentially least harmful and potentially most beneficial.

Predicting prognosis in acute alcoholic hepatitis

There is an urgent need for better instruments to identify which patients with potentially life-threatening liver disease are most likely to die in the near future. This aim has been achieved best for primary biliary cirrhosis and to a lesser extent fulminant hepatic failure (Shapiro *et al.*, 1979; Dickson *et al.*, 1989; O'Grady *et al.*, 1989). It has not been achieved to any practical degree in acute or chronic alcoholic liver disease. Acute alcoholic hepatitis poses particular prognostic problems. Many of these patients improve on withdrawal of alcohol, a fact which makes predicting prognosis extremely difficult (Chedid *et al.*, 1991). Maddrey and coworkers described a discriminant function derived retrospectively from a trial of corticosteroid therapy in acute alcoholic hepatitis. The revised discriminant function is calculated as follows: 4.6 (prothrombin time – control time) + serum bilirubin (mg/dl), and values greater than 32 indicate a high risk of early mortality (Carithers *et al.*, 1989). The discriminant function has been used in clinical trials of corticosteroids in acute alcohol hepatitis (Carithers *et al.*, 1989; Ramond *et al.*, 1992) and in those studies it clearly identified a high risk group of patients. In the placebo arm of Carithers' study, 11 of 31 high risk patients died within 28 days of enrollment. Similarly, in Ramond's study of high risk acute alcoholic hepatitis patients, 15 of 29 subjects who received placebo died by day 66. The practical problems which arise when considering patients with acute alcoholic hepatitis for liver transplant result from an inability to recognize patients who will recover with supportive care, which might include corticosteroid use. Unfortunately, in this crucial dilemma, the discriminant function does not help.

Predicting prognosis in alcoholic cirrhosis

When considering patients with chronic alcoholic liver disease, this issue is not so much determining which patient will recover but rather recognizing which patient is going to deteriorate to the point of requiring transplantation and when this will happen. The best established prognostic instrument is the Child–Turcotte classification in which five parameters were selected empirically as indicative of worsening hepatic dysfunction and therefore prognosis (Conn, 1981). The clinical parameters chosen were serum bilirubin, serum albumin, encephalopathy, ascites and nutritional status. Subsequently Pugh *et al.* (1973) modified this system by substituting prothrombin time for nutritional status and giving each parameter a points score (Table 4.2).

The Child–Turcotte–Pugh score is simple to use and especially valuable when stratifying patients within clinical studies. It also performs well against tests of integrated liver function, such as the aminopyrine breath test (Villeneuve *et al.*, 1986), or the more complex combined clinical prognostic scores derived by Cox regression analysis of prospective data (Christensen *et al.*, 1984). The Toronto group developed a complex clinical index which, while giving slightly more accurate prognostic data, is cumbersome and has not found widespread acceptance (Orrego *et al.*, 1983). Recently, attempts have been made to combine tests of integrated function (MEGX (monoethylglycinexylidide) test) and the Child–Turcotte–Pugh score with promising results (Oellerich *et al.*, 1991). Nonetheless, at the time of writing, clinical judgment based on Child–Turcotte–Pugh seems the best available prognostic method for patients with established chronic liver disease. With this approach it is possible to recognize advanced disease but not possible to be very accurate about estimated life span. An episode of spontaneous bacterial peritonitis carries a particularly poor prognosis, with more than 50% of individuals dead at 6 months in one series (Tito *et al.*, 1988).

The decision to place a patient on the transplant waiting list is made after consideration of the prognosis based on clinical parameters exemplified by the

Table 4.2. *Child–Turcotte–Pugh score*

	Child–Turcotte–Pugh score		
Points	1	2	3
Encephalopathy	None	1, 2	3, 4
Ascites	Absent	Slight	Moderate
Bilirubin (mg/dl)	1–2	2–3	> 3
Albumin (g/dl)	> 3.5	2.8–3.5	< 2.8
Prothrombin time (s. prolonged)	1–4	4–6	> 6
Primary biliary cirrhosis			
Bilirubin (mg/dl)	1–4	4–10	> 10

Grading (total score): 1–6: A; 7–9: B; 10–15: C.

Child–Turcotte–Pugh score. Specific features of decompensation such as intractable ascites requiring frequent paracentesis, recurrent variceal hemorrhage despite maximal medical therapy or an episode of spontaneous bacterial peritonitis may be indications for placement on the list. Finally, the ability of the patient to function is often an important consideration. We, therefore, inquire about lassitude, the requirement for daytime naps and the ability to work outside or within the home.

Prognostic factors predicting poor postoperative outcome

In addition to considering what factors indicate an increasing chance that a patient will die before a transplant becomes available, we and others have attempted to determine what preoperative clinical parameters predict outcome after transplantation surgery. In a retrospective review of 229 liver allograft recipients at the University of Michigan, severity of liver disease, as shown by Child–Turcotte–Pugh class, and preoperative creatinine level were significantly associated with higher mortality (Baliga *et al.*, 1992). The highest hospital mortality rate (32.6%) was observed in patients who were in the intensive care unit immediately before transplantation. The association of elevated creatinine levels with greater mortality was also observed by Cuervas-Mons *et al.* (1986). These data, along with those on prognosis for alcoholic liver disease reviewed above, indicate that the greatest chance for successful transplantation and the least chance for deterioration while awaiting transplantation occurs when patients with established liver disease are placed on the waiting list early rather than late in their disease course. At the same time, we try to delay listing while the patient's own liver can support a reasonable degree of day-to-day activity. A rule of thumb, albeit one not always adhered to, is 'a patient who can work, can wait for a liver transplant'. As mentioned earlier, the increasing unpredictability of a patient's waiting time make these deliberations fraught with difficulties.

Management of alcoholic liver disease

A comprehensive review of all aspects of the medical and surgical management of alcoholic liver disease is not appropriate here but specific therapies as they relate to liver transplantation are discussed.

Perhaps the most difficult clinical dilemma in patients with decompensated alcoholic liver disease is determining whether or not acute alcoholic hepatitis is going to resolve with medical therapy. As discussed in the section on prognosis, there are no good methods to distinguish between the patients who will respond to medical management and those who will not respond. Recently corticosteroids have enjoyed a new vogue (Carithers *et al.*, 1989; Imperiale and McCullough, 1990; Ramond *et al.*, 1992). Some, but not all, studies suggest that their benefits only occur in patients with encephalopathy. Although all recent studies exclude patients with renal failure, sepsis or active gastrointestinal hemorrhage, it appears that corticosteroids are worth trying in carefully selected patients with acute alcoholic hepatitis.

Patients with decompensated liver disease awaiting liver transplantation are at risk of developing spontaneous bacterial peritonitis. Prophylaxis against spontaneous bacterial peritonitis is worthwhile because in addition to the risks that it will precipitate death, an episode of peritonitis will cause the patient to be removed from the transplant waiting list for 4–10 days while effective treatment is given. Patients with ascites in which the albumin content is low or who have had a previous episode of variceal hemorrhage are at greatest risk of spontaneous bacterial peritonitis. Norfloxacin (400 mg daily) has been shown to significantly reduce the incidence of spontaneous bacterial peritonitis in patients with a history of at least one episode of spontaneous bacterial peritonitis or a high risk of a first episode (Gines *et al.*, 1990; Soriano *et al.*, 1991). It is probable that other quinolones would also be effective.

Prophylaxis against acute variceal hemorrhage can also be attempted in patients with end-stage liver disease. The risk of variceal hemorrhage is related to the severity of liver disease (as shown by Child–Pugh class), the size of varices and the presence on the varices of longitudinal red markings – so-called red wale marks (North Italian Endoscopic Club, 1988). Beta-adrenergic antagonists are effective in reducing the frequency of both recurrent bleeds and mortality in cirrhotic patients who have already bled from varices (Hayes *et al.*, 1990). The data are conflicting on the value of beta-blockade in patients with varices who have not bled (Hayes *et al.*, 1990; Poynard *et al.*, 1991; De Franchis *et al.*, 1991; Van Ruiswyk and Byrd, 1992). It is our practice to use endoscopy all prospective candidates for liver transplant who have clinical signs of portal hypertension and place patients at high risk of a first bleed on beta-blockade with propranolol even though not all studies support this course (De Franchis *et al.*, 1991). Prophylactic sclerotherapy for patients with varices which have not had a first bleed is not favored at present and may even be hazardous in alcoholic cirrhotics (Veterans Affairs Cooperative Variceal Sclerotherapy Group, 1991). The same view is probably true for elastic band ligation of varices as a prophylactic measure, although this has not been studied.

What is the role of liver transplantation in the management of patients who have bled from esophageal varices? At the University of Michigan we have taken a view similar to that of Bismuth *et al.* (1990) that patients with active bleeding should be controlled and then evaluated electively. Bismuth advises that among the patients who need more definitive therapy, Child–Turcotte–Pugh class A patients should receive a reduced-size portocaval shunt, Child–Turcotte–Pugh class C patients should be transplanted and Child–Turcotte–Pugh class B patients should be considered for shunt or transplant on a case by case basis. The emergency management of acute variceal bleeding will not be reviewed here except to say that most authorities would not favor proceeding to transplantation while a patient is hemodynamically unstable and therefore a risk for active hemorrhage. Emergency sclerotherapy, vasopressin and nitroglycerine, balloon tamponade, somatostatin and esophageal transection have been introduced into the armamentarium for control of active variceal hemorrhage (Burroughs *et al.*, 1989, 1990). It is worth noting that not all acute upper gastrointestinal hemorrhage related to portal hypertension arises from esophageal varices. Gastric varices, portal hypertensive gastropathy and occasionally duodenal varices can all cause upper gastrointestinal hemorrhage which is life threatening and difficult to control. Recently, Ring *et al.* (1992) have perfected a transjugular technique for insertion of an intrahepatic portocaval shunt that may remain patent for months. This method, called transjugular intrahepatic portosystemic shunt or TIPS, appears to be highly effective in controlling acute and chronic hemorrhage and holds particular promise of providing 'a bridge to transplantation'.

Table 4.3. *Clinical features in 99 patients with alcohol-related liver disease assessed for liver transplantation*

		Unsuitable for transplantation				
	Suitable for transplantation	Too well or suitable for other therapy	Too ill	Patient refused	Psychiatrically unsuitable	Total
Number of patients	45	17	19	1	17	99
Males	29	7	13	0	11	60
Females	16	10	6	1	6	39
Age (median) in years	44	37	52		45	
Range (years)	30–65	34–60	18–67		16–59	
Psychiatric evaluation	45	13	10	1	11	80
Dependent alcohol abuse[a]	39	11	6	1	9	66
Non-dependent alcohol abuse[a]	6	2	4	0	2	14
Duration of abstinence (months)						
Median	12	12	8		6	
Range	0–170	1–72	0–60		0–72	
Child's class						
A	0	5	0	0	1	6
B	12	7	1	0	3	23
C	33	5	18	1	13	70

[a] Defined according to DSM-III-R classification.

Malnutrition is very common in patients with alcoholic liver disease and indeed its presence may have some prognostic significance (Conn, 1981; Mendenhall *et al.*, 1986). Studies in patients with acute and chronic alcoholic liver disease have shown that protein dietary supplementation may improve clinical and biochemical parameters (Mezey *et al.*, 1991; Kearns *et al.*, 1992). It is probable that careful supplemental protein administration may benefit alcoholic patients awaiting transplantation although this has not been formally tested.

Outcome of the transplant selection process

In our review of 99 alcoholic patients who underwent liver transplant evaluation between 1985 and 1989 we found that 45 (43%) were considered suitable candidates and underwent transplantation (Lucey *et al.*, 1992*a*). In this section I will concentrate on the 54 (57%) candidates who were considered unsuitable. Their clinical details are shown in Table 4.3.

Seventeen patients were considered too well for transplantation or suitable for other therapy as shown in Figure 4.6. Their actuarial survival at 12 and 18 months was 93%. Thereafter, there was a sharp decline in survival to 59% at 24 months. This indicates that while we were accurate about predicting short-term survival, this prediction became less accurate after 18 months. The reasons for this decline are not clear. Many of these patients had been returned to their referring physicians for follow-up care. It is possible that the patients and/or their physician believed that the evaluation having been completed there was no need for continuing contact with the transplant center. It is possible that some patients returned to active drinking. Prospectively gathered data are not available on this point. The data make clear that in patients with chronic liver disease, consideration for liver transplantation is a dynamic rather than static process. Patients considered too well for transplantation should be referred again to a transplantation center when their clinical circumstances indicate decompensation and a change in prognosis.

Nineteen patients (20%) were considered medically unsuitable. These patients reflect the outcome of pursuing the second requirement of medical assessment as outlined at the beginning of this chapter, namely to search for medical conditions which would preclude successful transplantation. Twelve of 17 candidates were considered to be poor operative risks because of sepsis, acute ventilatory failure, acute alcoholic hepatitis or severe cardiac failure. Five patients were not selected because of hepatoma and one each because of aplastic anemia and caranoma of the lung. As shown in Figure 4.6, survival was very

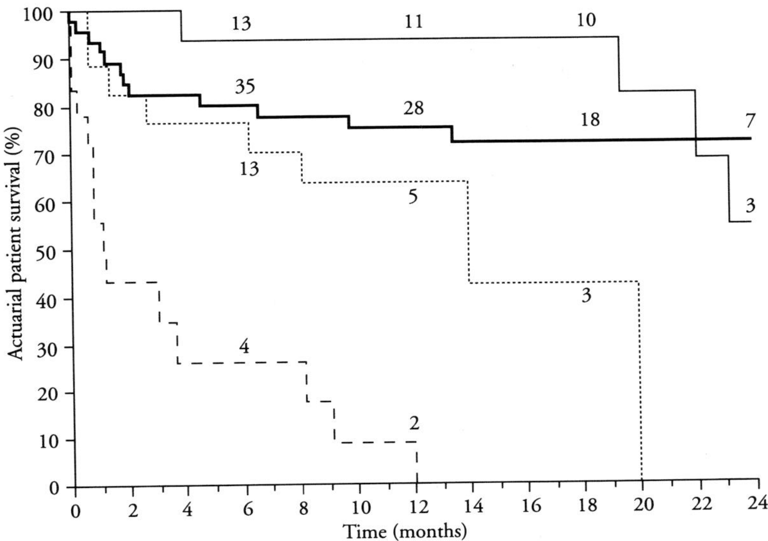

Figure 4.6. Actuarial survival curves in alcoholic patients undergoing liver transplantation or not selected for transplantation according to reason for non-selection. (▬) Transplanted. (——) Too well, not transplanted. (······) Psychiatric, not transplanted. (– – –) Too ill, not transplanted. Explanation of the categories is given in the text. Numbers shown in relation to each line represent the patients at risk at each time point. Reproduced from Lucey *et al.* (1992*a*), with permission.

poor in this group. Less than 50% of patients not selected because they were 'too ill' survived 1 month after referral, and all were dead or censored by 12 months.

Finally, there were 17 patients not selected on psychiatric grounds, i.e. a poor prognosis for abstinence. This group was similar to the transplanted group in age, sex and Child's class and thus was analagous to a control group. As shown in Figure 4.6, survival was significantly better in transplanted alcoholics than in alcoholics denied transplantation on psychiatric grounds: survival at 18 months was 73% vs 43%, respectively. In the absence of a controlled trial these data constitute the best evidence that liver transplantation is an efficacious treatment for decompensated alcoholic liver disease (see Chapter 1 for a more detailed discussion of the ethical issues of controlled trials of transplantation versus other forms of therapy).

References

Alexander, J.F., Lischner, M.W. and Galambos, J.T. (1971). Natural history of alcoholic hepatitis. II. The long-term prognosis. *American Journal of Gastroenterology*, **56**, 515–25.

Arria, A.M., Tarter, R.E., Starzl, T.E. and Van Thiel, D.H. (1991). Improvement in cognitive functioning of alcoholics following orthotopic liver transplantation. *Alcoholism, Clinical Experimental Research*, **15**, 956–62.

Baliga, P., Merion, R.M., Turcotte, J.G., Ham, J.M, Henley, K.S., Lucey, M.R., Schork, A., Shir, Y. and Campbell, Jr., D.A. (1992). Preoperative risk factor assessment in liver transplantation. *Surgery*, **112**, 704–11.

Bassett, M.L., Halliday, J.W. and Powell, L.W. (1986). Value of hepatic iron measurements in early hemochromatosis and determination of the critical iron level associated with fibrosis. *Hepatology*, **6**, 24–9.

Belli, L., Baticci, F., Belli, L.S., De Carlis, L., Del Favero, E., Donato, F., Makowka, L., Mazzaferro, V., Minola, E., Romani, F., Rondinara, G., Teperman, L. and Van Thiel, D. (1989). Reappraisal of surgical treatment of small hepatocellular carcinomas in cirrhosis: Clinicopathological study of resection or transplantation. *Digestive Diseases and Sciences*, **34**, 1571–5.

Bismuth, H., Adam, R., Mathur, S. and Sherlock, D. (1990). Options for elective treatment of portal hypertension in cirrhotic patients in the transplantation era. *American Journal of Surgery*, **160**, 105–10.

Bonkovsky H.L., Hawkins M., Steinberg K., Hersh T., Galambos J.T., Henderson J.M., Millikan W.J. and Galloway J.R. (1990). Prevalence and prediction of osteopenia in chronic liver disease. *Hepatology*, **12**, 273–80.

Borowsky, S.A., Stomre, S. and Lott, E. (1981). Continued heavy drinking and survival in alcoholic cirrhotics. *Gastroenterology*, **80**, 1405–9.

Brechot, C., Berthelot, P., Callard, P., Carnot, F., Courouce, A., Duhamel, G., Nalpas, B. and Tiollais, P. (1982). Evidence that hepatitis B virus has a role in liver-cell carcinoma in alcoholic liver disease. *New England Journal of Medicine*, **306**, 1384--6.

Burroughs, A.K., Hamilton, G., Phillips, A., Mezzanotte, G., McIntyre, N. and Hobbs, K.E.F. (1989). A comparison of sclerotherapy with staple transection of the esophagus for the emergency control of bleeding from esophageal varices. *New England Journal of Medicine*, **321**, 857–62.

Burroughs, A.K., McCormick, P.A., Hughes, M.D., Sprengers, D., D'Heygere, F. and McIntyre, N. (1990). Randomized, double-blind, placebo-controlled trial of somatostatin for variceal bleeding. *Gastroenterology*, **99**, 1388–95.

Carithers, Jr., R.L., Herlong, H.F., Diehl, A.M., Shaw, E.W., Combes, B., Fallon, H.J. and Maddrey, W.C. (1989). Methylprednisolone therapy in patients with severe alcoholic hepatitis. *Annals of Internal Medicine*, **110**, 685–90.

Charness, M.E., Simon, R.P. and Greenberg, D.A. (1989). Ethanol and the nervous system. *New England Journal of Medicine*, **321**, 442–54.

Chedid, A., Mendenhall, C.L., Gartside, P., French, S.W., Chen, T., Rabin, L. and the VA Cooperative Study Group. (1991). Prognostic factors in alcoholic liver disease. *American Journal of Gastroenterology*, **86**, 210–16.

Christensen, E., Schlichting, P., Fauerholdt, L., Gluud, C., Andersen, P.K., Juhl, E.,

Poulsen, H., Tygstrup, N. and The Copenhagen Study Group for Liver Diseases (1984). Prognostic value of Child–Turcotte criteria in medically treated cirrhosis. *Hepatology*, **4**, 430—5.

Colombo, M., De Fazio, C., De Franchis, R., Del Ninno, E., Di Carol, V., Dioguardi, N., Donato M.F., Sangiovanni, A. and Tommasini, M. (1991). Hepatocellular carcinoma in Italian patients with cirrhosis. *New England Journal of Medicine*, **325**, 675–80.

Compston J. (1986). Hepatic osteodystrophy: vitamin D metabolism in patients with liver disease. *Gut*, **27**, 1073–90.

Conn, H.O. (1981). A peek at the Child–Turcotte classification. *Hepatology*, **1**, 673–6.

Cuervas-Mons, V., Millan, I., Gavaler, J.S., Starzl, T.E. and Van Thiel, D.H. (1986). Prognostic value of preoperatively obtained clinical and laboratory data in predicting survival following orthotopic liver transplantation. *Hepatology*, **6**, 922–7.

Davies, S.E., Alexander, G.J.M., Aldis, P.M., Chaggar, K., O'Grady, J.G., Portmann, B.C. and Williams, R. (1991). Hepatic histological findings after transplantation for chronic hepatitis B virus infection, including a unique pattern of fibrosing cholestatic hepatitis. *Hepatology*, **13**, 150–7.

De Franchis, R., Primignani, M., Arcidiacono, P.G., Rizzi, P.M., Vitagliano, P., Vazzoler, M.C., Arcidiacono, R., Rossi, A., Zambelli, A., Cosentino, F., Caletti, G., Brunati, S., Battaglia, G. and Gerunda, G. (1991). Prophylactic sclerotherapy in high-risk cirrhotics selected by endoscopic criteria. *Gastroenterology*, **101**, 1087–93.

Diamond T., Stiel D., Lunzer M., Wilkinson M. and Posen S. (1989). Ethanol reduces bone formation and may cause osteoporosis. *American Journal of Medicine*, **86**, 282–8.

Diamond T., Stiel M., Lunzer, M., Wilkinson M., Roche J. and Posen, S. (1990). Osteoporosis and skeletal fractures in chronic liver disease. *Gut*, **31**, 82–7.

Di Bisceglie, A.M. (1991). Treatment of hepatocellular carcinoma. *Hepatology* , **13**, 802–4.

Dickson, E.R., Grambsch, P.M., Fleming, T.R., Fisher, L.D. and Langworthy A. ((1989). Prognosis in primary biliary cirrhosis: model for decision making. *Hepatology*, **10**, 1–7.

Diehl, A.M., Goodman, Z. and Ishak, K.G. (1988). Alcohol-like liver disease in non-alcoholics, a clinical and histologic comparison with alcohol-induced liver injury. *Gastroenterology*, **95**, 1056–62.

Feray, C., Samuel, D., Thiers, V., Gigou, M., Pichon, F., Bismuth, A., Reynes, M., Maisonneuve, P., Bismuth, H. and Brechot, C. (1992). Reinfection of liver graft by hepatitis C virus after liver transplantation. *Journal of Clinical Investigation*, **89**, 1361–5.

Franco, D., Bouzari, H., Capussotti, L., Dellepiane, M., Grange, D., Kemeny, F., Meakins, J. and Smadja, C. (1990). Resection of hepatocellular carcinomas, results in 72 European patients with cirrhosis. *Gastroenterology*, **98**, 733–8.

Frezza, M., DiPadova, C., Pozzato, G., Terpin, M., Baraona, E. and Lieber, C.S. (1990) High blood alcohol levels in women: the role of decreased gastoric alcohol dehydrogenase activity and first pass metabolism. *New England Journal of Medicine*, **322**, 95–9.

Geller, G., Bone, L.R., Levine, D.M., Mamon, J.A., Moore, R.D. and Stokes, E.J. (1989). Knowledge, attitudes, and reported practices of medical students and house staff regarding the diagnosis and treatment of alcoholism. *Journal of the American Medical Association*, **261**, 3115–20.

Gines, P., Quintero, E., Arroyo, V., Teres, J., Bruguera, M., Rimola, A., Caballeria, J., Rodes, R., and Rozman, C. (1987). Compensated cirrhosis: natural history and prognostic factors. *Hepatology*, **7**, 122–8.

Gines, P., Rimola, A., Planas, R., Vargas, V., Marco, F., Almela, M., Forne, M., Miranda, M.L., Llach, J., Salmeron, J.M., Esteve, M., Marques, J.M., Jimenez De Anta, M.T., Arroyo, V. and Rodes, J. (1990). Norfloxacin prevents spontaneous bacterial peritonitis recurrence in cirrhosis: results of a double-blind placebo-controlled trial. *Hepatology*, **12**, 716–24.

Gorensek, M.J., Carey, W.D., Goormastic, M. and Vogt, D. (1990). A multivariate analysis of risk factors for cytomegalovirus infection in liver-transplant recipients. *Gastroenterology*, **98**, 1326–32.

Hayes, P.C., Davis, J.M., Lewis, J.A. and Bouchier, I.A.D. (1990). Meta-analysis of value of propranolol in prevention of variceal hemorrhage. *Lancet*, **336**, 153–6.

Imperiale, T.F. and McCullough, A.J. (1990). Do corticosteroids reduce mortality from alcoholic hepatitis? A meta-analysis of the randomized trials. *Annals of Internal Medicine*, **113**, 299–307.

Ismail, T., Angrisani, L., Buckels, J.A.C., Elias, E., Gunson, B.K., Hubscher, S.G., McMaster, P. and Neuberger, J.M. (1990). Primary hepatic malignancy: The role of liver transplantation. *British Journal of Surgery*, **77**, 983–87.

Kearns, P.J., Young, H., Garcia, G., Blaschke, T., O'Hanlon, G., Rinki, M., Sucher, K. and Gregory, P. (1992). Accelerated improvement of alcoholic liver disease with enteral nutrition. *Gastroenterology*, **102**, 200–5.

Loft, S., Dossing, M. and Olesen, K.L. (1987). Increased susceptibility to liver disease in relation to alcohol consumption in women. *Scandinavian Journal of Gastroenterology*, **22**, 1251–6.

Lucey, M.R., Merion, R.M., Henley, K.S., Campbell, Jr., D.A., Turcotte, J.G., Nostrant, T.T., Blow, F.C. and Beresford, T.P. (1992*a*). Selection for and outcome of liver transplantation in alcoholic liver disease. *Gastroenterology*, **102**, 1736–41.

Lucey, M.R., Martin, P., Di Bisceglie, A., Rosenthal, S., Waggoner, J.G., Merion, R.M., Campbell, D.A., Nostrant, T.T. and Appelman, H. Recurrence of hepatitis B and delta hepatitis following orthotopic liver transplantation (1992*b*). *Gut*, **33**, 1390–6.

Martin, P., Armenti, V.T., Di Bisceglie, A.M., Jarrell, B.E., Maddrey, W.C., Moritz, M.J., Munoz, S.J., Rubin, R. and Waggoner, J.G. (1991). Recurrence of hepatitis C virus infection after orthotopic liver transplantation. *Hepatology*, **13**, 719–21.

Mendenhall, C.L., Tosch, T., Weesner, R.E., Garcia-Pont, P., Goldberg, S.J., Kiernan, T., Seeff, L.B., Sorrell, M., Tamburro, C., Zetterman, R., Chedid, A., Chen, T. and Rabin, L. (1986). VA cooperative study on alcoholic hepatitis II: prognostic significance of protein-calorie malnutrition. *American Journal of Clinical Nutrition*, **43**, 213–18.

Mezey, E., Caballeria, J., Mitchell, M.C., Pares, A., Herlong, H.F. and Rodes, J. (1991).

Effect of parenteral amino acid supplementation on short-term and long-term outcomes in severe alcoholic hepatitis: a randomized controlled trial. *Hepatology*, **14**, 1090–6.

Nishiguchi, S., Kobayashi, K., Kuroki, T., Monna, T., Otani, S., Sakurai, M., Seki, S., Shikata, T., Yamamoto, S. and Yabusako, T. (1991). Detection of hepatitis C virus antibodies and hepatitis C virus RNA in patients with alcoholic liver disease. *Hepatology*, **14**, 985–9.

Veterans Affiars Cooperative Variceal Sclerotherapy Group (1991). Propphylactic sclerotherapy for esophageal varices in men with alcoholic liver disease. *New England Journal of Medicine*, **324**, 1779–84.

O'Carroll, R.E., Hayes, P.C., Ebmeier, K.P., Dougall, N., Murray, C., Best, J.J.K., Bouchier, I.A.D. and Goodwin, G.M. Regional cerebral blood flow and coquitive function in patients with chronic liver disease. (1991) *Lancet*, **337**, 1250–3.

O'Grady, J.G., Alexander, G.J.M., Hayllar, K.M. and Williams, R. (1989). Early indicators of prognosis in fulminant hepatic failure. *Gastroenterology*, **97**, 439–45.

O'Grady, J.G., Calne, R.Y., Polson, R.J., Rolles, K. and Williams, R. (1988). Liver transplantation for malignant disease. *Annals of Surgery*, **207**, 373–9.

Oellerich, M., Burdelski, M., Lautz, H.-U., Binder, L. and Pichlmayr, R. (1991). Predictors of one-year pretransplant survival in patients with cirrhosis. *Hepatology*, **14**, 1029–34.

Olthoff, K.M., Busuttil, R.W., Goldstein, L.I., Millis, J.M., Ramming, K.P. and Rosove, M.H. (1990). Is liver transplantation justified for the treatment of hepatic malignancies? *Archives of Surgery*, **125**, 1261–8.

Orrego, H., Blendis, L.M., Blake, J.E., Kapur, B.M. and Israel, Y. (1979). Reliability of assessment of alcohol intake based on personal interviews in a liver clinic. *Lancet*, ii, 1354–6.

Orrego, H., Israel, Y., Blake, J.E. and Medline, A. (1983). Assessment of prognostic factors in alcoholic liver disease: Toward a global quantitative expression of severity. *Hepatology*, **3**, 896–905.

Pares, A., Barrera J.M., Bruguera, M., Caballeria, J., Caballeria, L., Castillo, R., Ercilla, G. and Rodes, J. (1990). Hepatitis C virus antibodies in chronic alcoholic patients: Association with severity of liver injury. *Hepatology*, **12**, 1295–9.

Porayko, M.K., Wiesner, R. H., Hay, J.E., Krom, R.A.F., Dickson, E.R., Beaver, S. and Schwerman L. (1991). Bone disease in liver transplant recipients: incidence, timing, and risk factors. *Transplantation Proceedings*, **23**, 1462–5.

Powell, E.E., Cooksley, G.E., Halliday, J.W., Hanson, R., Powell, L.W. and Searle, J. (1990).

The natural history of non-alcoholic steatohepatitis: a follow-up study of forty-two patients for up to 21 years. *Hepatology*, **11**, 74–80.

Powell, E.E., Pender, M.P., Chalk, J.B., Parkin, P.J., Strong, R., Lynch, S., Kerlin, P., Cooksley, W.G., Cheng, W. and Powell, L.W. (1990). Improvement in chronic hepatocerebral degeneration following liver transplantation. *Gastroenterology*, **98**, 1079–82.

Powell, W.J. and Klatskin, G. (1968). Duration of survival in patients with Laennec's cirrhosis. Influence of alcohol withdrawal and possible effects of recent changes in general management of the disease. *American Journal of Medicine*, **44**, 406–20.

Poynard, T., Cales, P., Pasta, L., Ideo, G., Pascal, J.-P., Pagliaro, L., Lebrec, D. and The Franco-Italian Multicenter Study Group (1991). Beta-adrenergic-antagonist drugs in the prevention of gastrointestinal bleeding in patients with cirrhosis and esophageal varices. *New England Journal of Medicine*, **324**, 1532–8.

Pugh, R.N.H., Murray-lyon, I.M., Dawson, J.L., Pietrony, M.C. and Williams, R. (1973). Transection of the esophagus for bleeding esophageal varices. *British Journal of Surgery*, **60**, 649–54.

Ramond, M.-R., Poynard, T., Rueff, B., Mathurin, P., Theodore, C., Chaput, J.-C. and Benhamou, J.-P. (1992). A randomized trial of prednisolone in patients with severe alcoholic hepatitis. *New England Journal of Medicine*, **326**, 507–12.

Ring, E.J., Lake, J.R., Roberts, J.P., Gordon, R.L., LaBerge, J.M., Read, A.E., Sterneck, M.R. and Ascher N.L. (1992). Using transjugular intrahepatic portosystemic shunts to control variceal bleeding before liver transplantation. *Annals of Internal Medicine*, **116**, 304—9.

Samuel, D., Arulnaden, J.L., Benhamou, J.P., Bismuth, A., Bismuth, H., Brechot, C., Mathieu, D. and Reynes, M. (1991). Passive immunoprophylaxis after liver transplantation in HBsAG-positive patients. *Lancet*, **337**, 813–15.

Shapiro, J.M., Smith, H. and Schaffner, F. (1979). Serum bilirubin: a prognostic factor in primary biliary cirrhosis. *Gut*, **20**, 137–40.

Shindo, M., Cheung, L., Cristiano, K., Di Bisceglie, A.M., Feinstone, S.M., Hoofnagle, J.H. and Shih, W.K. (1991). Decrease in serum hepatitis C viral RNA during alpha-interferon therapy for chronic hepatitis C. *Annals of Internal Medicine*, **115**, 700–4.

Sorenson, T.I.A., Bentsen, K.D., Christoffersen, P., Eghoje, K., Hoybye, G. and Orholm, M. (1984). Prospective evaluation of alcohol abuse and alcoholic liver injury in men as predictors of development of cirrhosis. *Lancet*, **ii**, 241–4.

Soriano, G., Guarner, C., Teixido, M., Such, J., Barrios, J., Enriques, J. and Vilardell, F. (1991). Selective intestinal decontamination prevents spontaneous bacterial peritonitis. *Gastroenterology*, **100**, 477–81.

Soterakis, J., Resnick, R.H. and Iber, F.L. (1973). Effect of alcohol abstinence on survival in cirrhotic portal hypertension. *Lancet*, **ii**, 65–7.

Stratta, R.J., Cushing, K.A., Donovan, J.P., Duckworth, R.M., Langnas, A.N., Li, S., Markin, R.S., Pillen, T.J., Reed, E.C., Shaefer, M.S., Shaw, Jr., R.W., Wood, R.P. and Woods, G.L. (1991). Successful prophylaxis of cytomegalovirus disease after primary CMV exposure in liver transplant recipients. *Transplantation*, **51**, 90–7.

Tarter, R.E., Switala, J., Arria, A., Plail, J. and Van Thiel, D.H. (1990). Subclinical hepatic encephalopathy. Comparison before and after orthotopic liver transplantation. *Transplantation*, **50**, 632–7.

North Italian Endoscopic Club for the Study and Treatment of Esophageal Varices (1988). Prediction of the first variceal hemorrhage in patients with cirrhosis of the liver and esophageal varices. A prospective multicenter study. *New England Journal of Medicine*, **319**, 983–9.

Tito, L., Rimola, A., Gines, P., Llach, J., Arroyo, V. and Rodes, J. (1988). Recurrence of spontaneous bacterial peritonitis in cirrhosis: frequency and predictive factors. *Hepatology*, **8**, 27–31.

Tzakis, A.G., Cooper, M.H., Dummer, J.S., Ragni, M., Starzl, T.E. and Ward, J.W. (1990). Transplantation in HIV+ patients. *Transplantation*, **49**, 354–8.

Urbano-Marquez, A., Estruch, R., Grau, J.M., Mont, L., Navarro-Lopez, F. and Rubin, E. (1989). The effects of alcoholism on skeletal and cardiac muscle. *New England Journal of Medicine*, **320**, 409–15.

Van Ruiswyk, J. and Byrd, J.C. (1992). Efficacy of prophylactic sclerotherapy for prevention of a first variceal hemorrhage. *Gastroenterology*, **102**, 587–97.

Van Thiel, D.H., Carr, B.I., Yokoyama, I., Iwatsuki, S. and Starzl, T.E. (1991). Liver transplanation as a treatment of hepatocellular carcinoma. In *Etiology, Pathology and Treatment of Hepatocellular Carcinoma in North America*, 1st edn, eds E. Tabor, A.M. Di Bisceglie and R.H. Purcell, pp. 309–15. Houston: Gulf Publishing Company.

Villeneuve, J.-P., Infante-Rivard, C., Ampelas, M., Pomier-Layrargues, G., Huet, P.-M. and Marleau, D. (1986). Prognostic value of the aminopyrine breath test in cirrhotic patients. *Hepatology*, **6**, 928–31.

Wright, H.I., Gavaler, J.S. and Van Thiel, D.H. (1992*a*). Preliminary experience with α-2b-interferon therapy of viral hepatitis in liver allograft recipients. *Transplantation*, **53**, 121–4.

Wright, T.L., Donegan, E., HSU, H.H., Ferrell, L., Lake, J.R., Kim, M., Combs, C., Fennessy, S., Robert, S.J.P., Ascher, N.L. and Greenberg, H.B. (1992*b*) Recurrent and acquired hepatitis C viral infection in liver transplant recipients. *Gastroenterology*, **103**, 317–22.

Zakim, D., Boyer, T.D. and Montgomery, C. (1989). Alcoholic liver disease. In *Hepatology, A Textbook of Liver Disease*, 2nd edn, eds, D. Zakin and T.D. Boyer pp. 821–68. Philadelphia: W.B. Saunders Company.

Note added in press:

Recently, both Hoofnagle *et al.* and Marcellin *et al.* have reported that careful administration of alpha interferon to cirrhotics with HBV infection occasionally produces spectacular improvements (Hoofnagle *et al.*, 1993; Marcellin *et al.*, 1993). Unfortunately, this therapeutic approach is associated with considerable risks and does not appear to prevent transmission of HBV to the allograft (Marcellin *et al.*, 1993; Lucey, 1993).

Hoofnagle, J.H., Di Bisceglie, A.M., Waggoner, J.G. and Park, Y. (1993). Interferon alfa for patients with clinically apparent cirrhosis due to chronic hepatitis B. *Gastroenterology*, **104**, 1116–21.

Lucey, M.R. (1993). Liver Transplantation for hepatits B infection – the art of the possible. *Hepatology* (in press).

Marcellin, P., Samuel, S., Areias, J., Loriot, M.A., Arulnaden, J.L., Gigon, M. and David, M.F. (1993). Pretransplantation interferon treatment and recurrence of HBV infection after liver transplantation for hepatitis B related end-stage liver disease. *Hepatolgy* (in press).

CHAPTER FIVE

OUTCOME OF LIVER TRANSPLANTATION FOR ALCOHOL-RELATED LIVER DISEASE

ROBERT M. MERION

General considerations

The earliest attempts at liver transplantation were undertaken in the 1960s by Thomas Starzl in Denver, Colorado and Sir Roy Calne in Cambridge, England. The pioneering efforts of these two surgeons (and their courageous patients) demonstrated that a liver allograft could be successfully transplanted in humans in the orthotopic position following removal of the patient's own diseased organ. Unfortunately, the first recipients were poor candidates by modern standards and the early reported results were disappointing (Starzl *et al.*, 1963; Williams, 1968). Requirements for successful organ preservation were poorly understood and logistically unattainable before the development of criteria for the diagnosis of brain death and the resultant acceptance of mechanically ventilated, heart beating cadaver donors. Immunosuppressive therapy was still in its infancy, allograft rejection was difficult to diagnose and reversal of established rejection was infrequently attained.

Fortunately, major advances occurred in each of these areas over the ensuing 25 years. Patient and graft survival have increased as a result of better patient selection, of improved surgical technique, the development of more reliable technology for organ preservation and major advances in critical care medicine. There have been significant strides in the understanding of transplantation immunology and new immunosuppressive agents (especially cyclosporine) have been developed. By 1983, a Consensus Development Conference sponsored by the National Institutes of Health concluded that liver transplantation should not be considered experimental and it was noted that 'patients who are judged likely to abstain from alcohol and who have established clinical indicators of fatal outcomes may be candidates for transplantation. Only a small proportion of alcoholic patients with liver disease would be expected to meet these rigorous criteria' (Anonymous, 1984). The assessment of abstinence prognostication is examined in detail elsewhere in this volume and will not be covered further here. The establishment of mortality markers in alcoholic patients is covered in Chapter 4 (medical suitability for liver transplantation). The perception that remains is that alcoholic patients might be unsuitable candidates for transplantation because of extrahepatic organ system dysfunction and that survival following transplantation would be poor.

Surgical technique and intraoperative management

Improvements in surgical technique have led to standardization of the operative procedure for liver transplantation and many of these advances have been of particular relevance to alcoholic recipient (Starzl and Demetris, 1990). The method now used by virtually all liver transplant programmes involves three major steps. The recipient's damaged liver is dissected free from its peritoneal attachments. At this point, the diseased organ is disconnected from its vascular connections and removed, leaving the patient completely anhepatic. The routine use of venovenous bypass during the anhepatic phase of the operation has greatly reduced the incidence of intraoperative hemodynamic instability and postoperative renal dysfunction (Griffith, *et al.*, 1985). This technique involves the placement of heparin-bonded cannulae into the lower vena cava and splanchnic side of the portal venous circulation to maintain venous return from the lower extremities, kidneys, intestines and spleen during the anhepatic phase of the procedure when the vena cava and portal vein are clamped. This is particularly important for recipients with a history of alcohol abuse or alcoholism who are at increased risk of cardiovascular morbidity from alcoholic cardiomyopathy, kidney dysfunction from associated preoperative renal insults and excessive hemorrhage from portal hypertension. The donor liver is implanted after native hepatectomy is completed. The vascular anastomoses are usually constructed in the following order: suprahepatic inferior vena cava, infrahepatic inferior vena cava, hepatic artery and portal vein. The donor liver is revascularized on completion of the vascular anastomoses. Biliary reconstruction (usually a choledochocholedochostomy) completes the reconstructive phase of the operation. Following establishment of hemostasis the abdomen is closed and the patient is taken to the surgical intensive care unit for postoperative management.

During the operative procedure, alcoholic recipients are at especial risk of developing cardiorespiratory instability at the time of revascularization when hydrogen ions, potassium and any retained preservative solution are released into the central venous circulation from the newly vascularized graft. Inotropic and chronotropic pharmacological support are frequently required. In addition to the cardiodepressive effects of revascularization, vasoactive effects in the setting of pulmonary arteriovenous shunts seen frequently in association with chronic liver disease may result in markedly increased pulmonary arterial pressure, increased airway pressures, and resultant impairment of oxygenation (Stoller, *et al.*, 1990). This may be catastrophic in alcoholic patients with pre-existing systemic hypoxemia if it is not anticipated and expeditiously treated.

The incremental risk of a previous portasystemic shunting performed for bleeding gastroesophageal varices is unknown. Alcoholic liver disease is by far the most common diagnosis among patients in North America who have undergone portasystemic shunts but these patients have until recently represented only a small proportion of liver transplant recipients. As an expanding population of patients with alcoholic cirrhosis is considered for transplantation, however, increasing numbers of alcoholic patients who have undergone shunt surgery for uncontrolled variceal hemorrhage will become liver transplant candidates. This may be offset, in part, by the recent development of the transjugular intrahepatic portasystemic shunt (TIPS) procedure. This angiographic technique has been utilized in patients who have variceal hemorrhage refractory to conventional means of non-operative control (endoscopic sclerotherapy, pharmacological intervention and esophageal balloon tamponade) but who are poor candidates for surgical portasystemic decompression. Such patients have been successfully 'bridged' to liver transplantation (LaBerge *et al.*, 1991). To assess the splanchnic venous anatomy, mesenteric arteriography is always performed as part of the transplant evaluation in post-shunt patients. Standard end-to-end anastomosis of the donor and recipient portal veins is performed if the main recipient portal vein is patent. Portal vein thrombectomy is successful if thrombosis has occurred recently but in some cases a bypass graft from the superior mesenteric vein is required using a conduit of donor iliac vein. Patients who develop portal vein sclerosis after shunting may also require venous grafting using iliac vein procured from the organ donor. These maneuvers add technical complexity to the operative procedure but with experience we and others (Brems *et al.*, 1989; Mazzaferro *et al.*, 1990; AbouJaoude *et al.*, 1991) have found that carefully selected patients do as well as previously shunted non-alcoholic recipients.

Postoperative management and immunosuppression

Routine postoperative management consists of several days of mechanical ventilation as part of a 7–10 day stay in the intensive care unit. Total transplantation hospitalization time averages about 4–5 weeks, during which time surgical recovery occurs, the return of gastrointestinal motility and the resumption of oral alimentation occur and immunosuppressive therapy is initiated. Prophylactic immunosuppression consists of an induction course of anti-lymphoblast globulin and maintenance therapy with cyclosporine, azathioprine and corticosteroids. Patients with stable immunologic courses are enrolled in a steroid withdrawal program after one year to avoid the consequences of long-term corticosteroid administration. At the time of writing, it is unclear what effect the advent of newer immunosuppressive agents (FK506, brequinar, rapamycin, mycophenolate mofetil, prostaglandins and deoxyspergualin) will have on this regimen.

Analysis of early postoperative graft function has demonstrated that liver function tests (serum transaminases, serum bilirubin and prothrombin time) are not significantly different when alcoholic recipients are compared with adult non-alcoholic patients. This suggests that the physiologic milieu encountered by the liver allograft in alcoholic recipients is not unfavorable to good graft function in the early postoperative phase. Similarly, there is no significant difference in the incidence or severity of rejection episodes (Table 5.1). This suggests that alcoholic recipients tolerate immunosuppressive therapy and argues against any clinically important persistence of the immunodepressive effects of alcohol as these recipients did not encounter a greater number of bacterial or fungal infections in the post-transplant period (Astry *et al.*, 1983).

Outpatient follow-up after hospital discharge is frequent during the first 3–6 months post-transplant. Surgical morbidity is common during this time, infections and other complications of immunosuppressive therapy may be seen and rejection may be diagnosed. Recipients are expected to attend the outpatient clinic as often as twice a week until their course is felt to be stable,

Table 5.1. *Allograft rejection following orthotopic liver transplantation occurring in 56 alcoholic liver transplant recipients and 56 case-matched non-alcoholic recipients*

	Alcoholic	Non-alcoholic	*p* value
Rejection (% patients)	27	36	NS
Episodes of rejection/patient	0.4 ± 0.8	0.7 ± 1.4	NS

Source: McCurry *et al.* (1992).

at which point the interval between visits is gradually lengthened and their general care is returned to the patient's referring physician.

The importance of patient compliance with a rigorous post-transplant inpatient management plan cannot be overemphasized. Liver transplant recipients must assume progressive responsibility for their care and develop a detailed understanding of a highly individualized medication regimen, including immunosuppressive therapy. Following an uncomplicated postoperative course, patients are taught the various aspects of their transplant aftercare and are instructed in the proper dosing and administration of medications. Recipients are given verbal as well as written information and materials to assist them in alerting the medical staff to untoward developments during the completion of the transplant hospitalization and during lifetime follow-up as an outpatient.

Understanding and compliance with a highly complex and demanding medical regimen is often difficult for the 'average recipient'. While difficult to quantify, alcoholic patients as a group appear to require an additional measure of attention from the transplant team in order to successfully assume these responsibilities. The incremental time and effort expended, especially by the social work and nursing staff, is rewarded by an uncommonly high level of interest and cooperation from the majority of alcoholic recipients in comparison to medical and surgical therapy other than transplantation extended to such patients.

Patient and graft survival

Before 1984, liver transplant recipients with a history of alcoholism were reported to have poor short and long-term survival. In recent years, however, data from large centers have demonstrated similar success rates for alcoholic and non-alcoholic recipients (Kumar, *et al.*, 1990; Bird, *et al.*, 1991; Lucey, *et*

Table 5.2. *Resource utilization by alcoholic and non-alcoholic patients undergoing orthotopic liver transplantation*

	Patient		
	Alcoholic	Non-alcoholic	*p* value
Days of mechanical ventilation[a]	10 ± 21	7 ± 12	NS
Days in intensive care unit[a]	13 ± 20	11 ± 13	NS
Hospital days[a]	33 ± 25	41 ± 34	NS
Number of readmissions/patient	1 ± 1	2 ± 2	N

[a] After operation.
Source: McCurry *et al.* (1992). The cohorts were chosen as described in the text and in Table 5.1.

interval (Figure 5.3). Actuarial graft survival among these same subgroups of patients is illustrated in Figure 5.4.

We have previously published results of a case control study of alcoholic and non-alcoholic adult liver transplant recipients (McCurry *et al.*, 1992). In that study 56 alcoholic patients who had undergone liver transplantation were compared with 56 non-alcoholic liver transplant recipients carefully matched for age, sex, Child–Pugh classification and transplant date as part of an attempt to discern whether transplantation for alcoholic cirrhosis entails excessive medical and surgical risk or resource utilization. In most respects, the alcoholic and non-alcoholic patients in the case control study were similar. The alcoholic recipients were more seriously ill, however, as reflected by a significantly higher proportion of recipients who required intensive care unit management up to the time of the transplant procedure. Serum bilirubin levels were significantly higher in the alcoholic recipients than in the non-alcoholic control patients as was the proportion of recipients with moderate or severe ascites (all $p < 0.05$).

Despite the increased severity of illness of the alcoholic recipients, operative results among the patients in the case control study demonstrated a remarkable similarity between alcoholic and non-alcoholic recipients. Blood transfusion requirements were virtually identical (approximately 30 units) and the rate of 30-day operative mortality was 9% in both groups. Actuarial patient survival at 1 year post-transplant was 75% for the alcoholic and 76% for the non-alcoholic recipients, respectively. Resource utilization as measured by the duration of mechanical ventilation, intensive care unit management, total hospitalization and rehospitalizations during the first post-transplant year was not significantly different between the two groups (Table 5.2).

These results clearly indicate that alcoholic recipients who undergo liver transplantation for end-stage alcoholic liver disease have an outcome that is as good as their non-alcoholic counterparts in every way. These findings strongly support transplantation as a medically appropriate therapy for such patients. One important caveat relates to the selection process by which these patients come to transplantation. Alcoholic patients with end-stage liver disease who are thought to be candidates for hepatic replacement should undergo a rigorous and uniformly applied medical, surgical and psychosocial evaluation at a center with experience in these areas (Beresford *et al.*, 1990). Without such a program, it is possible that surgical morbidity and mortality as well as long-term alcohol recidivism may be excessive, thus negating the beneficial effects of this life saving therapy and the squandering of limited donor organ resources.

Management of long-term medical problems

A comprehensive review of medical problems which occur in liver transplant recipients is beyond the scope of this text. Alcoholic and non-alcoholic recipients alike may experience renal dysfunction, hypertension, hyperuricemia, hypercholesterolemia and obesity after successful liver transplantation. Three long-term medical problems from which alcoholic patients are particularly at risk will be discussed in brief.

First, as described in Chapter 4, many patients with alcoholic cirrhosis are infected by hepatitis C at the time of transplantation. It has been clearly shown that patients who are viremic with hepatitis C virus at the time of transplantation nearly always experience infection of the allograft (Wright *et al.*, 1992). In some series up to 30% of recipients transplanted in the absence of evidence of hepatitis C infection acquire the virus in the perioperative period, presumably secondary to transfusion of infected blood or an infected donor organ. At present, it is difficult to predict the natural history of viral infection transmitted from a hepatitis C-positive donor. The infection is generally more indolent than post-transplant hepatitis B but may cause significant liver injury in some patients. It is not known whether the life cycle or pathologic potential of hepatitis C virus is modified by immunosuppressive agents.

Hepatitis B virus may also infect alcoholics. Current evidence suggests that patients with active viral replication at the time of transplantation are at highest risk of graft infection (Lucey *et al.*, 1992*b*). Liver allograft infection by hepatitis B virus may proceed very quickly and produce a histologic pattern which is unique to the transplanted liver (Figure 5.5). This phenomenon,

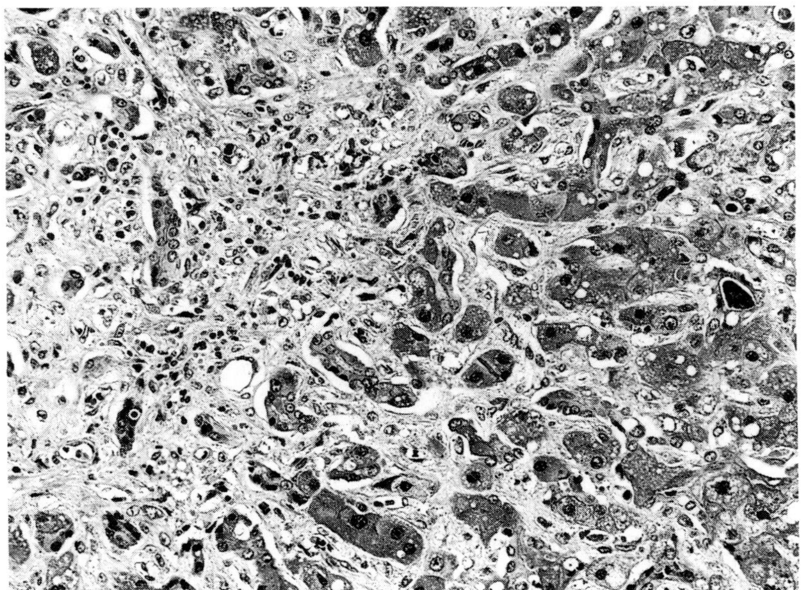

Figure 5.5. Light micrograph showing fibrosing cholestatic hepatitis in a liver allograft after transplantation for cirrhosis following hepatitis B virus infection. Reproduced with the permission of Lucey *et al.* (1992a).

called fibrosing cholestatic hepatitis, appears to be a consequence of the effect of immunosuppressive drugs, especially prednisone, on viral antigen production by infected hepatocytes (Davies *et al.*, 1991; Lucey *et al.*, 1992*b*). Fibrosing cholestatic hepatitis appears to portend a poor prognosis. Attempts have been made to prevent or retard the effects of recurrent viral hepatitis B in the allograft. The results of Samuel *et al.* (1991), using high volumes of high titer hepatitis B immune globulin, hold promise.

Second, alcoholic liver transplant recipients are at particular risk for recrudescence of *Mycobacterium tuberculosis.* In our own series, we have observed tuberculosis of the spine (Figure 5.6) and tuberculous pleural effusion in alcoholics who underwent liver transplant.

Third, alcoholic cirrhotics are often osteopenic and have a high risk of bony fractures (Bonkovsky, 1990; Diamond *et al.*, 1990). This is probably multifactorial in origin with liver disease, poor nutritional status and the inhibitory effect of ethanol on bone formation all playing a part (Compston, 1986; Diamond *et al.*, 1990). After solid organ transplantation such as kidney or liver allografting, there is a further rapid loss of bone mass (Julian *et al.*,

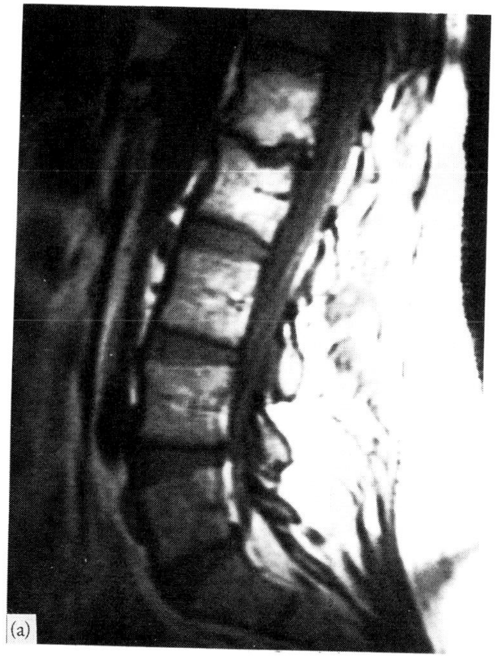

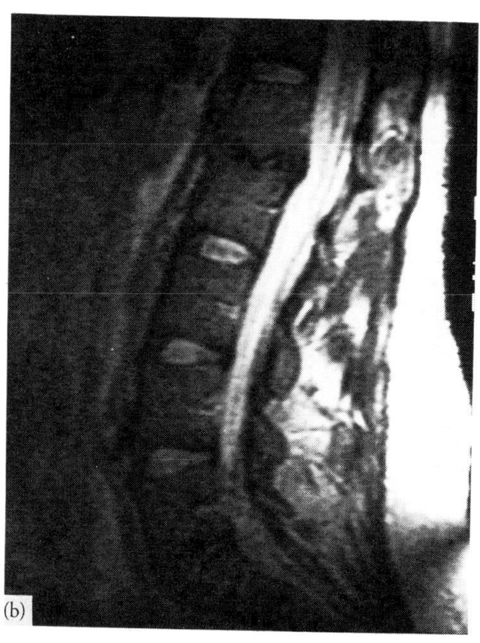

Figure 5.6. Magnetic resonance images of the lumbar spine in an alcoholic patient 16 months after liver transplantation. T_1 weighted (a) and T_2 weighted (b) images show loss of lumber L1–L2 disc space with distortion of the bony endplates. CT-guided aspiration of L1-L2 showed *Mycobacterium tuberculosis.* (Same as case 6.7, p. 107.)

1991; Porayko *et al.*, 1991). This effect has not been studied systematically in alcoholics undergoing liver transplantation but it seems reasonable to assume that bone loss may also occur after transplantation in alcoholic recipients. A putative major mechanism is the inhibitory effect of high dose glucocorticoids on bone formation. It is possible that post-transplant osteopenia and pathologic fractures might be less frequent in patients managed without long-term corticosteroids as part of the immunosuppressive regimen. At the University of Michigan, complete withdrawal of steroids has become a routine part of long-term management for liver transplant recipients whose course has been immunologically stable. More than 20 patients have been enrolled in a steroid withdrawal program and 14 have been completely weaned from prednisone. It is too early to predict whether steroid withdrawal alone will be associated with notable improvement in skeletal mineralization, however, as both cyclosporine and FK506 have been reported to produce osteopenia in rats (Katz and Epstein, 1992). It is likely, therefore, that postoperative bone disease will remain a source of morbidity in alcoholic and non-alcoholic recipients.

References

AbouJaoude, M.M., Grant, D.R., Ghent, C.N., Mimeault, R.E. and Wall, W.J. (1991). Effect of portasystemic shunts on subsequent transplantation of the liver. *Surgery, Gynecololgy and Obstetrics*, **172**, 215–19.

Anonymous (1984). National Institutes of Health Consensus Development Conference Statement: liver transplantation - 20–23 June 1983. *Hepatology*, **4**, 107S–110S.

Astry, C.L., Warr, G.A. and Jakab, G.J. (1983). Impairment of polymorphonuclear leukocyte immigration as a mechanism of alcohol-induced suppression of pulmonary antibacterial defenses. *American Review of Respiration Disease*, **128**, 113–17.

Beresford, T.P., Turcotte, J.G., Merion, R.M., Burtch, G., Blow, F.C., Campbell, D., Brower, K.J., Coffman, K., Modell, J.G. and Lucey, M. (1990). A rational approach to liver transplantation for the alcoholic. *Psychosomatics*, **31**, 241–54.

Bird, D.L.A., O'Grady, J.G., Harvey, F.A.H., Calne, R.Y. and Williams, R. (1990). Liver transplantation in patients with alcoholic cirrhosis: selection criteria and rates of survival and relapse. *British Medical Journal*, **301**, 15.

Bonkovsky, H.L., Hawkins, M., Steinberg, K., Hersh, T., Galambos, J.T., Henderson, J.M., Millikan, W.J. and Galloway, J.R. (1990). Prevalence and prediction of osteopenia in chronic liver disease. *Hepatology*, **12**, 273–80.

Brems, J.J., Hiatt, J.R., Klein, A.S., Millis, J.M., Colonna, J.O., Quinonas-Baldrich, W.J., Ramming, K.P. and Busuttil, R.W. (1989). Effect of a prior portasystemic shunt on subsequent liver transplantation. *Annals of Surgery*, **209**, 51–6.

Calne, R.Y. and Williams, R. (1968). Liver transplantation in man. I. Observations on technique and organization in five cases. *British Medical Journal*, **4**, 535–40.

Compston, J.E. (1986). Hepatic osteodystrophy: vitamin D metabolism in patients with liver disease. *Gut*, **27**, 1073–90.

Davies, S.E., Portman, B.C., O'Grady, J.G., Aldis, P.M., Chaggar, K., Alexander, G.J.M. and Williams, R. (1991). Hepatic histologic findings after transplantation for chronic hepatitis virus infection including a unique pattern of fibrosing cholestatic hepatitis. *Hepatology*, **13**, 150–7.

Diamond, T., Stiel, D., Lunzer, M., Wilkinson, M., Roche, J. and Posen, P. (1990). Osteoporosis and skeletal fractures in chronic liver disease. *Gut*, **31**, 82-87.

Griffith, B.P., Shaw, B.W., Hardesty, R.L., Iwatsuki, S. and Bahnson, H.T. (1985). Veno-venous bypass without systemic anticoagulation for transplantation of the human liver. *Surgery, Gynecology and Obstetrics*, **160**, 270–2.

Julian, B.A., Laskow, D.A., Dubovsky, J., Dubovsky, E.V., Curtis, J.J. and Quarles, L.D. (1991). Rapid loss of vertebral mineral density after renal transplantation. *New England Journal of Medicine*, **325**, 544–50.

Katz, I.A. and Epstein, S. (1992). Perspectives of posttransplantation bone disease. *Journal of Bone and Mineral Research*, **7**, 2.

Kumar, S., Stauber, R.E., Gavaler, J.S., Basista, M.H., Dindzans, V.J., Schade, R.R., Rabinovitz, M., Tarter, R.E., Gordon, R., Starzl, T.E. and Van Thiel, D.H. (1990). Orthotopic liver transplantation for alcoholic liver disease. *Hepatology*, **11**, 159.

LaBerge, J.M., Ring, E.J. and Lake, J.R., (1991). Transjugular intrahepatic portasystemic shunts: preliminary results in 25 patients. *Journal of Vascular Surgery*, **16**, 258–67.

Lucey, M.R., Graham, D.M., Martin, P., Di Bisceglie, A., Rosenthal, S., Waggoner, J.G., Merion, R.M., Campbell, D.A. and Appelman, H.D. (1992*a*). Recurrence of hepatitis B and delta hepatitis after orthotopic liver transplantation. *Gut*, **22**, 1390–6.

Lucey, M.R., Merion, R.M., Henley, K.S., Campbell, D.A., Turcotte, J.G., Nostrant, T.T., Blow, F.C. and Beresford, T.P. (1992*b*). Selection for and outcome of liver transplantation in alcoholic liver disease. *Gastroenterology*, **102**, 1736–41.

McCurry, K.R., Baliga, P., Merion, R.M., Ham, J.M., Lucey, M.R., Beresford, T.P., Turcotte, J.G. and Campbell, D.A. (1992). Resource utilization and outcome of liver transplantation for alcoholic cirrhosis - a case control study. *Archives of Surgery*, **127**, 772–7.

Mazzaferro, V., Todo, S., Tzakis, A.G., Stieber, A.C., Makowka, L. and Starzl, T.E. (1990). Liver transplantation in patients with previous portasystemic shunt. *American Journal of Surgery*, **160**, 111–16.

Porayko, M.K., Wiesner, R.H., Hay, J.E., Krom, R.A.F., Dickson, E.R., Beaver, S. and Schwerman, L. (1991). Bone disease in liver transplant recipients: incidence, timing, and risk factors. *Transplantation Proceedings*, **23**, 1462–5.

Samuel, D., Arulnaden, J.L., Benhamou, J.P., Bismuth, A., Bismuth, H., Brechot, C., Mathieu, D. and Reynes, M. (1991). Passive immunoprophylaxis after liver transplantation in HBsAG positive patients. *Lancet*, **337**, 813–15.

Scharschmidt, B.F. (1984). Human liver transplantation: analysis of data on 540 patients from four centers. *Hepatology*, **4**, 955.

Starzl, T.E. and Demetris, A.J. (1990). Development of the replacement operation. In *Liver Transplantation*, Starzl, T.E. and Demetris, A.J. (Eds), Year Book Medical Publishers, Chicago, pp. 3–41.

Starzl, T.E., Marchioro, T., VonKaulia, K., Hermann, G. and Brittain, R. (1963). Homotransplantation of the liver in humans. *Surgery, Gynecology andObstetrics*, **117**, 659–76.

Stoller, J.K., Moodie, D., Schiavone, W.A., Vogt, D., Broughan, T., Winkelman, E., Rehm, P.K. and Carey, W.D. (1990). Reduction of intrapulmonary shunt and resolution of digital clubbing associated with primary biliary cirrhosis after liver transplantation. *Hepatology*, **11**, 54–8.

Wright, T.L., Donegan, E., Hsu, H.H., Ferrell, L., Lake, J.R., Kim, M., Combs, C., Fennessy, S., Robert, S.J.P., Ascher, N.L. and Greenberg, H.B. (1992). Recurrent and acquired hepatitis C viral infection in liver transplant recipients. *Gastroenterology*, **103**, 317–22.

CHAPTER SIX

PSYCHIATRIC FOLLOW-UP CARE OF ALCOHOL-DEPENDENT LIVER GRAFT RECIPIENTS

THOMAS P. BERESFORD

Introduction

To understand the goals of follow-up care for alcohol-dependent transplant patients one must first understand the natural histories of the two conditions. As indicated earlier in this volume, the expected postoperative course is survival and return to premorbid function once the first few weeks have passed. Continuous improvement in hepatic functioning with concomitant recovery of function in the activities of daily life appears to be the outcome for most transplant recipients (Wolcott, 1990); current studies should provide further information. The natural history of alcoholism predicts a waxing and waning course over many years and some writers have compared it witho the course of other chronic illnesses such as diabetes mellitus or hypertension (Vaillant, 1983). With these courses in mind, the goals of follow-up psychiatric care are twofold: (1) the continued abstinence from ethanol both as an hepatotoxic

Table 6.3. *Any alcohol exposure in 25 dependent and 25 non-dependent recipients matched for sex and time since transplant*

	Dependent		Non-dependent	
Months	*n*	Alcohol exposure	*n*	Alcohol exposure
12–23	8	2	6	1
24–35	13	4	9	4
36–47	3	1	8	5
>48	1	0	2	2

alcohol dependence at preoperative evaluation and were accepted for transplantation only if they were considered to be at low risk for alcoholism relapse as determined by assessing the series of prognostic factors discussed in the previous chapter. A fixed period of preoperative sobriety was not required. Patients who did not survive for 6 months (n=13) were excluded as was one patient for whom the results of preoperative evaluation was not available. This left a group of 38 patients who were followed from 6 to 63 months after surgery with a mean of 36 months. Actuarially defined post-transplant abstinence from any alcohol exposure was 92% at 1 year and 74% at both 2 and 3 years. Clinically, five of the patients had suffered alcohol relapses that required medical hospitalization: one of these died from graft rejection owing to poor compliance with the anti-immune medicines while another suffered from severe allograft dysfunction at the time of the study and from the same cause. A third patient suffered intermittent bouts of pancreatitis, the fourth a cellulitis in one lower extrememity and the fifth was admitted for treatment of acute alcohol withdrawal. Seven additional patients experienced limited drinking relapses for brief periods but did not require hospitalization. Cox proportional hazards regression demonstrated that neither the length of preoperative abstinence nor a scale that attempted to quantify the prognostic factors at baseline reliably predicted subsequent alcohol use in this highly selected group of patients. This study concluded that, over the long term, the majority (69%) of selected alcohol-dependent recipients may abstain completely whereas an additional minority (18%) may experience brief relapses that do not result in liver graft injury or otherwise require hospitalization, in part the result of attentive long-term follow-up care. A small minority (13%) appear to return to pathologic drinkig leading to hospitalization and infrequently to death. These data argue for continued allocation of liver grafts to carefully selected alcohol-dependent candidates but they also point to the need to improve prognostic and follow-up methods.

The drinking relapse rate among alcoholic transplant recipients reported by most centers is significantly lower than that expected among non-selected groups of alcohol rehabilitation attenders. The best rates of abstinence among the latter reported in the literature are in the range of the 50–60%. (Moos, 1990) Based on early data, this difference tentatively suggests that the combination of the transplant experience and those factors relating to long-term abstinence, all in a setting of selection for long-term good outcome, are probably effective. Only a larger number of patients, carefully selected and evaluated, along with well-defined control or comparison groups, will establish this as a reasonable conclusion.

Psychiatric conditions among alcohol-dependent liver graft recipients

Any surgery that is as profoundly invasive as a liver transplant procedure will necessarily carry with it a series of postoperative conditions and reactions. There are excellent guides available to the presentation, course and treatment of these conditions insofar as they are common to any major abdominal surgery (Hall, 1980; Cassem, 1991; Craven and Rodin, 1992). In what follows, we will focus on those conditions that, to the best of our present knowledge, appear unique to alcohol-dependent patients who receive a liver graft. Discussion of these conditions will necessarily be brief but we hope that it will alert clinicians to the occurrence of these phenomena.

Postoperative delirium and organic mental disorders

Several programs have reported the occurrence of delirium and related organic mental disorders among alcoholic liver recipients both informally and in the medical literature (Trzepacz *et al.*, 1989). No systematic studies, however, have confirmed the impression that these conditions occur more frequently among alcoholics than among non-alcoholics. From a phenomenologic point of view, there appear to be two types of brain disorder that can be classified as delirium.

The first of these is an acute delirium beginning in the immediate postoperative period. It is characterized by profound disorientation, confusion, inability to focus attention and, frequently, behavioral agitation, none of which can be attributed to specific organ failure as evidenced by other signs or symptoms or as measured by standard laboratory parameters. The following case provides a striking example of this form of delirium.

Case 6.3. This 37-year-old alcoholic female appeared acutely confused in the intensive care unit one day after her liver transplant. She had been free of alcohol for the previous 4 years. On examination she was awake and alert but with a fluctuating ability to attend to subjects of conversation. She could not recall her name. She intermittently fixed her attention on her hospital bracelet on which was written both her name and the name of the admitting clerk, a male. She was very puzzled by this and could not decide which of the two names was hers. She could not respond when the interviewer asked her what gender she was. She was not oriented to place or time and could not focus her attention long enough to perform mental status tasks. She was unable to comprehend that she had had major surgery. While she was emotionally labile, she was not physically agitated and did not attempt to leave the hospital bed or the intensive care unit. Her liver indices were normal as was her blood ammonia level. There were no focal findings. The CT scan of the head revealed no evidence of a mass or lesion.

Physicians may find a specific cause in only about half of delirium cases because of the relative non-specificity of the symptoms (Cassem, 1991). Effective clinical practice, therefore, should focus on the effort to rule out as many likely causes of delirium, such as liver or renal failure or a focal central nervous system lesion, that are related to the operative procedure, to medication or to both. As an example, our experience has included two cases of stroke following the transplant procedure, perhaps in relation to the vasocontricting properties of cyclosporine In most cases specific physical or laboratory indicators are absent and the delirium must be treated symptomatically. In the case 6.3, the psychiatrist prescribed an antipsychotic agent in a low dose, 1 mg of oral haloperidol given twice daily. The delirium cleared within 12 hours. The medication was stopped on the third day and there was no recrudescence of confusion or other delirious symptoms. This reversibility constitutes another prime characteristic of a delirium and should be expected in the vast majority of cases. Case 6.3 is also noteworthy for its remarkable severity: it is rare for delirious patients to suffer a confusion to the extent of not recognizing name and gender. Clinical experience suggests that graft recipients with a previous history of alcoholism may be more susceptible to delirium of this severity. Further systematic research must establish or refute this, however.

Part of the confusion seen in acute delirium involves an inability to locate oneself properly with respect to space and time. Another facet is the general inability to focus attention for more than brief periods. In the absence of these faculties, more complicated procedures, such as mathematical calculation or recent memory production, are very difficult to test. Consider the next case.

Case 6.4. This 62-year-old alcoholic male received a liver transplant followed by listlessness during post-surgical recovery that proceeded more slowly than for most patients. Two weeks after the operation a psychiatric consultant interviewed him and found him attentive, cooperative and cognizant of person, place and date. He could not recall any of four objects at 5 minutes, however, and was unable to calculate simple addition and subtraction or to recall his fund of knowledge. These were losses of function compared with a preoperative interview. He was prescribed thioridazine, 25 mg orally twice daily for 3 days. The patient's symptoms cleared remarkably over the next 2 days. At interview on the third day, the patient had only a vague recollection of the period since his surgery.

This case represents a second, less florid form of delirium, which we will term subacute delirium, occurring in the postoperative period. In subacute delirium, patients do not necessarily appear confused and are generally able to attend to a conversation for brief periods. When more difficult tasks, such as recent memory tests, calculations, tests of judgement or of fund of knowledge, are tested these patients either cannot perform them or do so in a very slow, laborious manner often not completing them. Emotional lability is often present and may be reported by the nursing staff. As in the case of acute delirium, brief treatment with very low doses of antipsychotic medication is remarkably effective in returning the impaired central nervous system to normal functioning. The potentially hepatotoxic effects of antipsychotic medications must always be kept in mind because the potential harm of a continuing delirious process that may result in patient injury or self-neglect generally outweighs the rare toxic effects at appropriately low doses. To minimize toxic risks further, most clinicians employ a brief, time-limited course of medication.

Another type of brain disorder occurs in the immediate postoperative period, is related to delirium and might be called an acute delusional episode. In such cases, the ability to focus one's attention and to locate one's self in place and time have been preserved. So too have some or most higher cortical functions such as calculating ability, memory recall, fund of knowledge and the ability to derive abstract meanings. Emotional propriety, however, may be disturbed and delusional productions become apparent at the clinical interview. In one case, the delusional material was subtle.

Case 6.5. The psychiatrist was called to see this 57-year-old white male alcoholic 7 days after liver transplant because the transplant staff felt that he was not responding with appropriate energy and enthusiasm to his post-operative care. At interview he presented a nearly clear cognitive mental status but impressed the interviewer with a bland, almost detached emotional expression. After questioning, the patient described to the psychiatrist the belief that he was now beyond time, having passed out of human existence to the supernatural world. The patient felt very uneasy about this belief and was not reassured by the psychiatrist's reorienting statements. This patient received 25 mg of oral thioridazine twice daily for the next four days with complete remission of his symptoms. As in case 6.4, he recalled very little of his post-transplant experience once he had regained his faculties.

In other cases, however, the post-operative delusions may be more florid and present in ways more reminiscent of a delirious process.

Case 6.6. This 45-year-old alcoholic male with no prior history of psychosis underwent an uneventful liver transplant procedure but was noted to be somewhat sedated during the first 24 hours after surgery. By the third day he appeared neither confused nor disoriented. On the fifth postoperative day, while sitting in his room he had a visual hallucination in which he saw himself as on a great movie screen: he was leaving the hospital in the company of his family and wearing a particularly stylish blue suit that had come to him from Europe. He became agitated after this vision, feeling that God had allowed him to look forward into the events of time. He told no one of this vision for 2 days.

One week after surgery he became angry at a nurse whom he believed was trying to hurt him. The psychiatrist was called and found an emotionally labile patient who was able to attend and to speak calmly. The patient recounted the visual hallucination for the first time but was unable to accept the idea that it might have been an hallucination rather than a supernatural experience. The patient calculated simple addition and subtraction problems and named four of the five last Presidents but could recall only two of four objects after 5 minutes. He reluctantly agreed to medication: 1 mg of haloperidol by mouth twice daily. After 4 days he developed an akathisia from the haloperidol and was switched to oral thioridazine, 25 mg twice daily. Two days later he developed a tremor from sharply rising cyclosporine levels; the tremor disappeared when the dose was reduced but after 1 week of thioridazine at this dose, the patient's symptoms were unchanged.

During a visit home he became emotionally labile and attempted to attack a family member. He was returned to the hospital. Thioridazine orally at 50 mg twice a day had no effect. The thioridazine was discontinued and a trial of lithium carbonate, 300 mg three times a day was begun which resulted in a blood level of 0.7 mEq/l. During the third week of his convalescence the patient reluctantly agreed to transfer to a psychiatric unit wherein this medication and progress could be monitored more closely. Over the next 2 weeks his symptoms gradually receded and he was discharged home.

In the absence of organ failure, one looks naturally to toxic causes as the basis for the different organic mental states presented in these cases. Each of the patients above received a daily dose of prednisone in the range of 20–35 mg, as well as the standard postoperative doses of cyclosporine. Prednisone, like other steroid compounds, has been shown to cause delirious or organic mental processes that resemble affective psychoses such as mania or depression. In general, however, in the absence of other confounding factors, the minimum dose of prednisone required for development of a toxic psychosis is thought to be in the range of 40 mg daily (Boston Collaborative Drug Surveillance, 1972). Most transplant patients receive less than this amount. At the same time the central nervous system side-effects of cyclosporine are well known (Lucey *et al.*, 1990; Craven, 1991). Its neurologic manifestations often serve as the clinical endpoint of dose titration. Cyclosporine alone, however, may not account for the deliria noted above; anecdotal experience with this medicine, used without prednisone in persons suffering severe dermatologic disease, suggests that it does not frequently result in a delirium or an organic mental state. It may be that the interaction of these two medications provides a synergistic effect resulting in a state that neither would necessarily cause alone.

At the same time, it is important to note that each of these cases occurred in a chronic alcoholic patient none of whom had a previous history of psychosis and among whom there was a wide range of intervals since last alcohol use. It may be that postoperative organic mental conditions occur more frequently or with greater severity in this patient population because of a previously impaired central nervous system, a fragility of a sort that may not come to light without the added stress of a toxic insult. Clinical research must tell us whether this is the case and lead us toward an understanding of the possible mechanisms involved.

Fortunately, even the most severe cases have responded to specific treatment or to the passage of time or both. In most instances, low dose antipsychotic medications represent the agents of choice. Lithium carbonate, reportedly effective against steroid-induced depressions or manic states (Falk *et al.*, 1979; Goggans *et al.*, 1983), may be considered a second-line agent. To the best of our experience, antidepressant medicines are probably not useful in this setting and benzodiazapine compounds have offered neither rationale nor evidence of effective use in these cases. Careful attention to mental status changes in the acute postoperative period followed by appropriate treatment when indicated offers our best, most clinically effective, management of delirious processes at the present time.

Postoperative pain

Although infrequent, postoperative pain may last beyond the first several days after surgery and, for some patients, evolve into a chronic pain condition. There are generally two obvious and immediate causes of postoperative pain: the surgery itself and reactions to the antiimmune medicines, most notably cyclosporine.

In the acute post-surgical period alcoholic persons, especially those who have a history of abuse of other drugs including opiates, may require more pain-killing medication than non-alcoholic or non-opiate abusing patients. These medications should be given for brief periods in doses required to control the pain and should be tapered and discontinued when they are no longer needed. Some patients may request opiate medicines beyond the acute recovery period. This may be in response to chronic abdominal pain owing to the surgery or to some other cause. Should this occur, careful evaluation is the first step as in the following case.

Case 6.7. This 34-year-old alcoholic woman complained of severe lower back pain radiating to her lower extremities. After an extensive evaluation, including magnetic resonance imaging, no cause for the pain could be found. The patient, who had had a history of both alcoholism and poly-drug dependence, asked for opiate medicines because they were the only agent that offered her relief from an excruciating pain. The psychiatrist was called to assess her 'drug seeking behavior'. At evaluation the patient stated her reluctance to use opiates because of her 6 years of 'clean time'. She was also, however, very frightened and powerless in the face of her pain. The psychiatrist could find no 'functional' cause for her behavior.

The attending surgeon reviewed the pain evaluation and repeated the physical examination. He found a trigger point for the pain in the lower spine. High-resolution tomograms of this area highlighted what appeared to be a possible abscess involving one of the spinal nerve roots. Needle aspiration brought forth fluid that grew the tubercle bacillus, the apparent residue of an old hip fracture from an automobile accident. Prompt institution of antitubercular medicines relieved this patient of her pain, as well as of her need or desire for opiate medicines. (See also Figure 5.6, p. 92.)

The possibility of addictive behavior among alcoholic patients should always be considered in a differential diagnosis and the above case points to the necessity for careful evaluation to allow for effective treatment. In most cases, however, chronic pain may persist through mechanisms that are not so definitively treatable. The best approaches to chronic pain have been well described elsewhere (Cassem, 1991) and will not be repeated here except to underline the point that chronic opiate or benzodiazapine preparations should be avoided in any chronic pain patient as often as possible. This is clearly the case with alcohol or other drug-dependent patients. There may be times, however, when this is not possible as in the following case.

Case 6.8. This 40-year-old white male was 7 years free of both alcohol and opiate drugs after an extensive history of dependence on both. Before his liver transplant he had had occasional severe migraine headaches which were amenable only to opiate medicines or to inactivity in a darkened room. Before surgery, the patient who was an active participant in Narcotics Anonymous, refused opiate drugs for his headaches and would isolate himself until they passed. Following liver transplant and daily cyclosporine, he began noticing headaches that occurred without warning and with greater severity than before surgery. They occurred as often as three or four times weekly and lasted from 4 to 8 hours. When the headache pain became severe, he used a codeine preparation prescribed by the surgeons. After several months of this, he was referred to the psychiatrist who found no evidence of tolerance or escalating use. In the patient's words, 'If these don't work, there's nothing between me and the pain. I use as few as I can'.

Untreated headaches caused this patient to miss his work, denying him his livelihood. After trials of several non-opiate medicines met with little success, the patient and the transplant team arrived at a plan for continued intermittent use of opiate medicines to control the pain. Issues of chronic pain are often difficult and are likely to be a continuing part of liver transplant practice, especially among alcoholic or drug dependent patients. Much remains to be learned about the application of standard approaches to chronic pain for patients in this relatively new physiologic environment.

Drug substitution

One of the truisms for those trained in the addictions is that a person who is addicted to one drug is very likely to be or to become addicted to another or perhaps to all other drugs of abuse. This may more appropriately describe the population of poly-drug abusers than most alcoholic patients and many would argue that addiction to one substance, such as alcohol, does not necessarily predispose towards addiction to another substance and that the addiction to a second substance must be demonstrated by clinical evidence. The idea of potential universal addiction, however, would predict that when one substance, such as alcohol, is given up as in the case of the liver transplant recipient, that vulnerable patients may replace it with another addictive substance. Indeed, members of transplant teams around the USA have noted cases such as this one.

Case 6.9. This 33-year-old alcoholic male engaged in an active social life in his pre-transplant days. He spent many of his evenings and weekends in the company of others who drank heavily and occasionally used illegal substances. His own pattern of alcoholism was clear and was shadowed by a pattern of occasional marijuana use that did not reach the proportions of dependence. Following his transplant and recuperative period, he gave up alcohol completely but occasionally smoked marijuana. By the second year post-transplant he reported to his physicians that he often used marijuana in place of alcohol during social functions. A psychiatric evaluation revealed an increased use of marijuana but no evidence of the other major symptoms of addiction. He presented no other history of drug use, including sedatives, stimulants or pain-killing preparations. The patient had never shown evidence of impairment of the liver graft. The psychiatrist joined the members of the transplant team in recommending against marijuana use.

Needless to say, this patient's behavior presented a difficult question for the transplant team. On the one hand, no one was comfortable with the patient's using marijuana, both for legal reasons as well as for their concerns that this alcoholic patient might become addicted to a new drug. On the other hand, there was no clinical evidence that his marijuana use was taking on the proportions of an addiction and, given his otherwise stable functioning, no indication that he should seek treatment. It was especially important to note that there was no cocaine use in this patient's history, as marijuana use frequently predicts resumption of cocaine use in those individuals who have been addicted to it. The resolution in this case was a mutual sense of unease between patient and team that resulted in follow-up by mutual consent. As these kinds of instances occur, it will become important to understand their nature, as well as their implications for long-term survival and organ functioning. The relative infrequency of such occurrences argues strongly for a multi-center study of such phenomena that would shed light on this clinical difficulty.

Postoperative depression

The process of the liver graft brings with it many changes in life. One natural reaction to change is a transient depression. In the survey of alcoholic and non-alcoholic transplant recipients mentioned above, we noted both the perception of a major change in life as well as the high frequency of depression in both patient groups. These are listed in Table 6.4.

These data suggest that the likelihood of depression lasting more than 1 month is higher among the alcoholic recipients (14%) than among the non-alcoholic recipients (5%) and that the latter approximates the rate of the major affective disorders in the general population. This may be useful as a clinical reminder but the numbers in this sample are too small for valid generalization and none of the patients presented evidence of a major affective disorder. Only further systematic research from several transplant centers will tell whether alcoholic liver graft recipients are more likely to be depressed than non-alcoholic recipients.

Table 6.4. *Liver transplant group comparisons: depression and change*

	Alcohol dependent (*n*=22)	Non-alcohol-dependent (*n*=39)
Any mental health problems ever	4	3
Mental health fair or poor at present	3	3
Felt depressed post-transplant	15	26
Depressed > 1 week	5	5
Depressed > 1 month	4	2
Feels fair or poor after transplant	3	10
Life changed after transplant	20	30
Family relationships	12	18
Better	10	15
Worse	2	3
Employment	7	18
Better	2	4
Worse	5	14
Finances	14	20
Better	0	1
Worse	14	19
Spiritual/religious issues (better only)	8	18

It is clear, however, that a particular form of depression can beset either group and that is the depression caused by continued cyclosporine/prednisone therapy. We noted above that this combination appears to be related to delirium in the acute postoperative phase. Experience suggests that it may also play a role in what may be termed an organically-induced depression that may present well after the acute hospitalization and recuperation from surgery. Here is a representative case.

Case 6.10. This 52-year-old non-alcoholic patient was referred by the transplant team for psychiatric evaluation of depression. The patient presented with complaints of feeling 'down' and 'weepy' with occasional difficulty in controlling his emotions in the presence of his family. He felt that his condition would never change and, at 14 months after his transplant, he began to wonder whether his mood would ever improve. He had not experienced any suicidal or homicidal thoughts or plans. He had had no delusions or hallucinations. His cognitive abilities were intact. He had no vegetative symptoms of depression such as early morning awakening or a diurnal mood variation. Asked to describe which of his symptoms gave him the greatest discomfort, he replied that it was his changeable mood. The psychiatrist prescribed 25 mg of thioridazine taken at bedtime. At return visit 2 weeks later, the patient reported a nearly complete reversal of his mood lability. Even his wife had commented on his improved outlook. The patient continued on this regimen for 1 month after which it was discontinued with no further report of symptoms.

This form of depression resembles clinical reports of 'prednisone depression' although the dose in this case was much lower: 12.5 mg daily in combination with cyclosporine. The patient tolerated a small dose of antipsychotic medicine given in a time limited fashion. Whether this might be better supplanted by another agent such as lithium carbonate with much less hepatotoxic risk must await further clinical study. In the meantime, it is most important for clinicians to differentiate this form of depression from major depressive disorder, requiring specific treatment through tricyclic antidepressant medications or electroconvulsive therapy, as well as from the dysthymic conditions that respond to an ongoing psychotherapeutic relationship. In this area of medicine as in most, proper diagnosis and specific treatment offer the best outcome.

Finally, there is another presentation of post-transplant depression that may be more frequent among some alcohol abusing patients. Recent attention in both the popular and scholarly literatures has focused on the long-term effects of childhood or adolescent sexual or physical abuse. For some who have undergone such experiences, alcohol abuse or dependence may play a role in maintaining a further 'adjustment' to life. In the absence of alcohol, a painful depression may occur resembling that seen in cases of post traumatic stress syndrome. This, in turn, may result in returning to alcohol or resorting to another agent of abuse. In most cases careful inquiry followed by appropriate psychotherapy and attention to abstinence behavior constitute a treatment of choice. Very little data exist on this topic generally and considerably less is available in the transplant setting. For now, clinicians should be aware of it and include it in the differential diagnosis.

References

Beresford, T. P., Schwartz, J., Wilson, D., Merion, M. and Lucey, M.R. (1992). The short-term psychological health of alcoholic and non-alcoholic liver transplant recipients. *Alcoholism: Clinical and Experimental Research*, **16**, 996–1000.

Boston Collaborative Drug Surveillance (1972). Acute adverse reactions to prednisone in relation to dosage. *Clinical Pharmacology and Therapeutics*, **13**, 694–8.

Cambpell, D.A., Beresford, T.P., Merion, R.M., Punch, J.D., Ham, J.M., Lucey, M.R., Baliga, P. and Turcotte, J.T. (1993). Alcohol use relapse following liver transplantation for alcoholic cirrhosis: long-term follow-up. Abstract, Proccedings of the American Society of Transplant Surgeons. Houston, Texas, 20–22 May, p. 131.

Cassem, E. H. (1991). *The MGH Handbook Of General Hospital Psychiatry.* St. Louis, Mosby-Yearbook

Craven, J.L. and Rodin, G.M. (1992). *Psychiatric Aspects Of Organ Transplantation.* Oxford, Oxford University Press

Craven, J. L. (1991). Cyclosporine-associated organic mental disorders in liver transplant recipients. *Psychosomatics*, **32**, 94–102.

Falk, W.E., Mahnke, M.D. and Poskanzer, M.D. (1979). Lithium prophylaxis of corticotropin- induced psychosis. *Journal of the American Medical Association*, **241**, 1011–12.

Goggans, F.C., Weisberg, L.J. and Koran, L.M. (1983). Lithium prophylaxis of prednisone psychosis: a case report. *Journal of Clinical Psychiatry*, **44**, 111–12.

Hall, R.C.W. (1980). *Psychiatric Presentations Of Medical Illness.* New York, Spectrum.

Kumar, S., Stauber, R. E., Gavaler, J. S., Batista, M. H., Dindzans, V. J., Schade, R. R., Rabinovitz, M., Tarter, R. E., Gordon, R. and Starzl, T. E. (1990). Orthotopic liver transplantation for alcoholic liver disease. *Hepatology*, **11**, 159–64.

Lucey, M. R., Kolars, J.C., Merion, R.M., Campbell, D.A., Aldrich, M. and Watkins, P.B. (1990). Cyclosporine toxicity at therapeutic blood levels and cytochrome P-450 IIIA. *Lancet*, **335**, 11–15.

Moos, R. M., Finney, J.W. and Cronkite, R.C. (1990). *Alcoholism Treatment .* New York, Oxford University Press.

Trzepacz, P. T., Brenner, R. and Van Thiel, D. (1989). A psychiatric study of 247 liver transplantation candidates. *Psychosomatics*, **30**, 147–53.

Vaillant, G. (1983). *The Natural History Of Alcoholism.* Cambridge, Mass., Harvard University Press.

Wolcott, D. L. (1990). Organ transplant psychiatry: psychiatry's role in the second gift of life. *Psychosomatics*, **31**, 91–7.

CHAPTER SEVEN

ETHICS, ALCOHOLISM AND LIVER TRANSPLANTATION

MARTIN BENJAMIN AND
JEREMIAH G. TURCOTTE

Introduction

Are alcoholic patients responsible for their end-stage liver disease (ESLD) in ways that other ESLD patients are not? If so, should this be a consideration in determining access to the limited supply of transplantable livers? Does justice require that non-alcoholic ESLD patients be given priority over alcoholic patients? Or does justice actually require that carefully selected, abstinent alcoholics be provided the same opportunity to receive a new liver as medically suitable non-alcoholic patients?

In what follows we identify and critically examine the three main positions on these and related questions. The first argues that patients whose ESLD is attributable to alcohol consumption should nearly always have a lower priority for receiving a new liver than patients whose ESLD is attributable to other factors. The second position maintains that carefully selected alcoholic patients should be allowed to compete equally with non-alcoholic patients for transplantable livers. The third position is a compromise between the first two. The fact that alcohol consumption is likely to have contributed to a carefully selected transplant candidate's ESLD should, on this view, be given some weight in allocation decisions but not so much that such candidates invariably have a lower priority than others.

Personal responsibility for liver failure

The claim that alcoholic ESLD patients are personally responsible for their disease and should, as a result, have a lower priority for receiving a new liver than other ESLD patients has been developed and defended by Moss and Siegler (1991). In what follows we outline their argument and critically assess it.

The argument

Until recently, alcoholic ESLD patients have, for medical reasons, constituted a relatively small proportion of transplant recipients. Liver transplantation in such patients was simply not very successful (Scharschmidt, 1984). Yet there is growing reason to believe that carefully selected alcoholic ESLD patients are likely to do quite well as transplant recipients. One report of liver transplantation in carefully selected alcoholics reveals 1-year survival rates comparable to those of non-alcoholic patients (Starzl *et al.*, 1988). Another report indicates the same for 2-year survival (Lucey *et a.l.*, 1992) Moreover, methods and criteria for distinguishing good from bad risks among alcoholic patients are becoming increasingly sophisticated and accurate (Beresford *et al.*, 1990; Lucey and Beresford, 1992; Lucey *et. al.*, 1992). As a result, a number – perhaps a very large number – of alcoholic ESLD patients may no longer be denied access to transplantation on medical grounds alone.

Alcohol consumption is responsible for more than 50% of ESLD amd the inclusion of carefully selected alcoholics in the pool of potential liver recipients is likely to place considerable strain on the already very limited supply of transplantable livers. If allowed to compete equally for access to transplantation, some alcoholic patients will certainly receive a liver before some non-alcoholic patients who will then die. Is this just or fair? Should those whose need for a new liver is attributable to heavy drinking be permitted to gain access to transplantation before, and in some cases at the expense of, those whose need for an organ is attributable to other causes?

A common argument for allowing medically suitable alcoholic patients to compete equally with non-alcoholics is that alcoholism, no less than ESLD, is a disease and that it is unjust to judge or withhold needed medical treatment from patients for reasons associated with a disease from which they suffer. Yet this line of reasoning, Moss and Siegler contend, misses the point. It is not alcoholism as such that is at issue, but rather the patient's failure to seek treatment for his or her alcoholism: 'Although alcoholics cannot be held responsible for their disease, once their condition has been diagnosed they can be held responsible for seeking treatment and for preventing the complications of [alcohol-related] ESLD' (Moss and Siegler, 1991, p. 1297).

Treatment for alcoholism, Moss and Siegler maintain, is widely available and reasonably effective:

> One comprehensive review concluded that more than two-thirds of patients who accept therapy improve. Another cited four studies in which at least 54% of patients were abstinent a minimum of 1 year after treatment. A recent study of alcohol-impaired physicians reported a 100% abstinence rate an average of 33.4 months after therapy was initiated. In this study, physician-patients rated Alcoholics Anonymous, the largest organization of recovering alcoholics in the world, as the most important component of their therapy (Moss and Siegler, 1991, p. 1296)

Treatment cannot be effective if it is not undertaken, and the decision to undertake treatment, they add, is a matter of personal responsibility. That this decision is within the power of those suffering from alcoholism is borne out, Moss and Siegler argue, by the large numbers of alcoholics enrolled in and achieving some measure of success in various treatment programs.

Alcohol-related ESLD is the product of 10–20 years of heavy drinking. Given common knowledge about the many negative consequences of years of heavy alcohol consumption, the availability of effective treatment programs, and the scarcity of transplantable livers, alcoholics must accept some responsibility for developing ESLD if, over this period, they have made no reasonable effort to seek and obtain treatment aimed at keeping their disease in remission. The fact that they are responsible for the development of their ESLD in a way that, for example, patients with congenital biliary atresia or primary biliary cirrhosis are not, legitimates differential treatment. Again, what is at issue is not alcoholism, but rather the alcoholic's (moral) failure to seek and obtain treatment for it, treatment that could have prevented the development of ESLD.

A fundamental principle of justice requires similar treatment for relevantly similar cases. For example, it is unjust to treat similarly ill patients differently simply because one patient is black and the other white, or because one patient is male and the other female. Differences in skin color or sex are not in themselves morally relevant with respect to determining treatment for similarly ill patients. The difference between alcoholic and nonalcoholic ESLD patients is, Moss and Siegler contend, an ethically relevant consideration in determining access to liver transplantation. Unlike skin color and gender, heavy drinking is something an alcoholic patient could have done something about; he or she could have sought and obtained treatment that may have been successful in preventing the need for liver transplantation. Thus, there is an ethically relevant difference between those whose ESLD is attributable to alcohol and other ESLD patients. This difference, under conditions of scarcity, requires different treatment. Individuals who have had absolutely no control over the development of their ESLD have a stronger claim to liver transplantation under conditions of scarcity than those who, if they had chosen, could have done something to prevent their ESLD. Similar treatment for ethically dissimilar cases constitutes, in this context, a grave injustice.

A related principle of justice requires holding individuals responsible for the effort they make in achieving certain ends. We rightly respect those who work hard to achieve commendable goals even if their efforts are not fully successful. We cannot commend those who make the effort to seek and obtain treatment for their illnesses without being prepared to criticize those who do not. Both types of response are related to the Kantian notion of respect for persons or autonomous choice. To respect an individual as a person is to respond to him or her in ways that are determined by the autonomous choices and efforts he or she has made. To respond in ways that systematically ignore or overlook an individual's choices or personal efforts is to fail to recognize and respect him or her as a self-determining being (Morris, 1968).

An additional ethical consideration, one based more on the principle of utility than on principles of justice, draws our attention to the public's perception of liver transplantation for alcoholic patients. Given the high cost of liver transplantation, together with the fact that this cost is partly borne by a public with a decidedly dim view of alcoholics and alcoholism, providing access to alcoholic patients might well lead to a decline in overall public support for liver transplantation to the detriment of all ESLD patients.

Thus, Moss and Siegler conclude, considerations of justice, fairness and utility require that patients whose ESLD results from heavy drinking should, under conditions of scarcity, have a lower priority for access to liver transplantation than patients whose ESLD is caused by factors entirely beyond their control. Patients whose ESLD is attributable to alcohol consumption should be eligible for transplantation only if there were no other patients who could benefit from an available donor liver. Non-alcoholic patients should, in other words, be given priority even over the most medically suitable alcoholic patients. The only exception should be for alcoholic ESLD patients who meet the following three conditions: they (1) had sought treatment for their heavy drinking, but (2) were unable, for reasons beyond their control, to obtain it, and (3) are now abstaining from alcohol and considered, after careful medical, psychiatric and social evaluation, good candidates for transplantation. Alcoholic patients meeting these conditions, and only those meeting them, may be allowed to compete equally with medically suitable non-alcoholic patients for the limited supply of transplantable livers.

Assessment of the argument

The foregoing argument suffers from a number of difficulties. First, it applies a double standard in singling out alcohol-related ESLD from among the many diseases in which patient behavior plays a causal role. Second, it presumes more knowledge about degrees of voluntariness than is actually warranted. Third, it is insensitive to the wide variety of cases in which alcohol may be a factor in the development of ESLD. Fourth, its single-minded emphasis on personal responsibility disregards the importance of other ethical values, particularly likelihood of success, in organ allocation. Finally, it underestimates the public's capacity to distinguish drunkenness and irresponsibly drunken behavior from alcoholism.

Double standard

A number of severe illnesses are attributable to patient conduct. Consider, for example, well known connections between lung cancer and smoking or between heart disease and overeating, sedentary lifestyle, smoking and a failure to take prescribed medication. Physicians repeatedly urge patients to refrain from or seek treatment for patterns of behavior that they know are likely to result in life threatening illnesses, the treatment for which is extremely costly. Yet patients who ignore such advice and succumb to the forewarned illnesses are invariably treated, and with no hesitation. Why, then, should alcoholic

ESLD patients be singled out for different treatment? Is this not arbitrary or discriminatory? It is difficult, in this light, to suppress the suspicion that it is actually prejudice against alcoholism, and not simply concerns about responsibility for illness, that drives the personal responsibility argument in the context of liver transplantation.

Moss and Siegler anticipate this objection and reply, first, by drawing a general distinction between absolute and relative scarcity and, second, by comparing liver with heart transplantation. Liver transplantation, they argue differs from many other expensive lifesaving therapies inasmuch as it requires a 'non-renewable, absolutely scarce resource', which distinguishes it from 'most other resources such as dialysis machines and ventilators, both of which are only relatively scarce' (Moss and Siegler, 1991). Dialysis machines and ventilators are only relatively scarce because their availability is a function of our willingness to purchase them. Were we willing to spend more money, we could readily increase the supply. The same is not true, however, about the scarcity of transplantable organs. Barring the development of artificial livers or successful xenografting, we cannot increase the limited supply of transplantable livers simply by 'throwing money' at the problem.

The distinction between absolute and relative scarcity becomes less significant, however, when, later in their paper, Moss and Siegler support the principle of *To each, treatment according to personal effort* by appealing to the need for overall health care rationing at the level of macro-allocation of resources (Moss and Siegler, 1991, p. 1297). Once a nation begins to ration health care, what was once only relatively scarce may, for all practical purposes, become absolutely scarce. Dialysis machines in the UK, for example, have been reported to be absolutely scarce as a result of explicit policy decisions made by the National Health Service (Aaron and Schwartz, 1984). The advent of health care rationing at the macro-level will, therefore, force Moss and Siegler to extend the personal responsibility argument to cases involving 'renewable' but perhaps very expensive resources that are limited by design. If they are prepared to do so, they must then address the wider, more general, far-reaching and extremely controversial implications of applying the personal responsibility criterion to all kinds of medical care. If they are not prepared to do so, they must explain why it is not arbitrary or discriminatory to apply this criterion only to alcohol-related ESLD.

Choosing to restrict themselves to considerations of absolute scarcity, Moss and Siegler then provide two arguments for distinguishing liver transplantation from heart transplantation, so as to avoid having to address the extent to which the need for heart transplantation is also, in a number of cases, partly self-induced. They argue, first, that the causal connection between, say smoking, overeating, sedentary life style, not taking prescribed medication and so on, and heart disease is less direct than the causal connection between heavy drinking and liver failure. They do not explain the moral relevance of this difference. Physicians are deeply concerned about the connection between smoking, overeating, sedentary life style, not taking prescribed medication, and so on and various other illnesses. Are we to conclude from Moss and Siegler's argument that they should be less concerned about these connections than about the connection between heavy drinking and ESLD? Moreover, the connection between alcoholism and ESLD is not as direct as they seem to suggest (Lucey and Beresford, 1992). The vast majority of alcoholics will not develop ESLD; and a significant percentage of those who develop alcoholic cirrhosis, many of them women, will neither be alcoholics nor have a genuine alcohol dependence. Moreover, it is in fact difficult in certain cases to determine whether cirrhosis has been caused by heavy drinking or by other factors (Lucey and Beresford, 1992).

These fuel the suspicion that the operative difference in many people's thinking is that alcohol consumption has been traditionally regarded as a vice whereas smoking, overeating, sedentary life style and so on have not. If this were so, however, the argument relies more heavily on shallow moralizing than on a genuine ethical difference.

Moss and Siegler's second argument for distinguishing heart from liver transplantation is that a history of alcohol abuse is a de facto contraindication for heart transplantation. But can this contraindication still be justified? That this is the case is one thing; that it ought to be the case is another. Perhaps those performing heart transplants need to undertake a more refined evaluation of candidates with a history of heavy drinking to determine which are likely to do well and which are not. Without demonstrable evidence that all former heavy drinkers in need of a new heart are bad risks, especially in the light of recent data about success rates in liver transplantation for carefully selected alcoholics, this may be based on little more than prejudice, intuition or outdated assumptions.

Considerations of scarcity and justice may eventually lead to rationing policies in which those individuals demonstrably responsible for their illnesses may not be entitled to customary treatment. If so, such policies must be applied to all illnesses for which individuals are relevantly responsible and not only to those illnesses bearing a moralistic taint. To do otherwise is to apply an arbitrary double-standard and to violate the principle of justice requiring similar treatment for similar cases.

Voluntariness

Can we say, with confidence, that an apparent failure to seek effective treatment for alcoholism has always been within each person's power? Moss and Siegler rely heavily on the self-help gospel preached by members of Alcoholics Anonymous and other such groups. These are often strong and admirable individuals who have done a remarkable job of lifting themselves by their own bootstraps. It takes nothing away from their accomplishments, however, to wonder whether all people at all stages of their lives are similarly capable; whether, that is, it is always within each person's power to take control of his or her drinking (or smoking, overeating, etc.) by enrolling in an effective treatment program. Most of us can, for example, recall performing wrongful or harmful acts in the past that we believe now we were, at those times, powerless to resist.

The point is that there are limits to what we can know about another's willpower and the degree of voluntariness of their actions. This should temper the temptation to make facile judgments about alcoholics' responsibility for seeking treatment for alcoholism, especially in a culture in which drinking is not only legal, but has been portrayed in films and television commercials as glamorous and sophisticated. The law does not prohibit heavy drinking and other aspects of the culture positively encourage it (Makela and Room, 1985). That some people, once they have been encouraged to begin drinking, may find it extremely difficult – perhaps, at certain stages of their lives, psychologically impossible – to stop should not be surprising. High-minded moralism with respect to such individuals is, at best, insensitive and, at worst, unjust.

Contingencies

The personal responsibility position places a premium on the availability of effective treatment. This, however, raises many questions. Are effective treatment programs available to all who might benefit from them? Are the most effective treatment programs also the most costly and, as a result, accessible only to the wealthy, the well-insured or, perhaps, the well-connected? Do all alcoholics have access to the sort of treatment programs available to wealthy celebrities, like Betty Ford and Kitty Dukakis, or to physicians? Medicare and Medicaid pay for transplantation but do they also pay for effective alcohol treatment? Is it possible that some individuals – perhaps those living in sparsely populated rural areas or in extremely poor and crowded urban areas or those in unique personal or family circumstances – would have no real access to effective alcohol treatment facilities until they are sick enough to be treated for severe liver failure? How should we respond to an individual whose heavy drinking began before becoming a teenager, when personal responsibility for the consequences of one's actions is not fully developed, and who, by the time he or she has developed the independent strength of will to seek effective treatment, has developed ESLD?

Towards the end of their paper, Moss and Siegler acknowledge that patients with alcohol-related ESLD who had not previously been offered therapy and who are now abstaining from alcohol could be eligible for liver transplantation. How are these individuals to be identified? Are physicians to hire private detectives to investigate their pasts? Is this a practical or attractive role for medicine to assume?

The point of these questions is to highlight a dilemma for the personal responsibility position. If it is justly applied, it must take account of an enormous number of complexities that will, among other things, require intrusive investigations on the part of physicians into the private lives of their patients. If on the other hand, one ignores these complexities, implementation of the personal responsibility is likely to involve numerous injustices.

Other values

The personal responsibility position gives non-alcoholics with ESLD a higher priority for receiving liver transplants than alcoholic patients. Priority, however, can be a matter of degree or it can be absolute. For Moss and Siegler it is largely absolute. Alcoholic patients are either in or out. If they were not previously offered treatment for their alcoholism or if there are no non-alcoholic recipients for available livers, they are in. Otherwise, they are categorically precluded.

This conclusion seems incompatible with the actual process for allocating transplantable livers, which is a computerized point system involving a number of important values and that operates by marking differences of degree. Candidates for particular livers are awarded a certain number of points for such factors a blood type (recipients with the same ABO type as the donor are awarded 10 points, those with compatible but not identical types are given 5 points, and those with incompatible types are given 0 points), time on the waiting list (10 points for those waiting longest with fewer points for those with shorter tenure) and degree of medical urgency (ranging from 24 points for the most urgent to 0 points for the least urgent).

Underlying this system for allocating livers are a multiplicity of values: utility or medical success (blood type compatibility), fairness (time on waiting list) and some combination of utility and fairness (degree of medical urgency). Yet adopting of the personal responsibility position would require over-riding all these other considerations in the case of alcoholic patients. For example a carefully selected, abstinent alcoholic who, with respect to a particular donor liver, might otherwise have received 10 points for ABO compatibility, 10 for time on the waiting list and 24 for urgency of need, would be passed over for a non-alcoholic patient receiving 0 points for ABO compatibility, 0 points for time on the waiting list and 12 for urgency of need (or such a patient could conceivably receive 10 for compatibility, 0 for time on the waiting list and 6 for degree of urgency). The wasteful consequences of the personal responsibility position in this case should make us pause.

Thus in allowing (alleged) personal responsibility for ESLD to 'trump' all other values involved in organ allocation, Moss and Siegler ignore other important values, especially those having to do with maximizing host and graft survival. No consideration seems to be given to the most effective use of a limited lifesaving resource under conditions of scarcity. Of two possible liver recipients, one of whom is likely to do much better than the other, the one with greater likelihood of medical success will, if he or she is a carefully selected abstinent alcoholic, be absolutely precluded from obtaining the organ because of a history of heavy drinking. Again, it is difficult not to suspect that shallow moralizing about the evils of drink has obscured a more complex, morally and medically sensitive understanding of the many values involved in organ allocation.

Public perception

Moss and Siegler buttress their justice-based arguments with considerations of utility. The public's negative view of alcoholism, they suggest, may lead to a lowering of support of liver transplantation in general if it learns that alcoholics come to constitute a significant portion of the recipient population. Thus, for the sake of preserving the greater good of the system of liver transplantation, they argue, we ought to give a higher priority to non-alcoholic candidates. The argument not only presumes that the public's inability to distinguish alcoholism from the deplorable consequences of drunken behavior, but it also, most unfortunately, reinforces it. At one point Moss and Siegler cite Mothers Against Drunk Driving and Students Against Drunk Driving to support their claim.

Drunk drivers are, we agree, a public menace but not all alcoholics are drunk drivers and not all drunk drivers are alcoholics. Identifying alcoholism with drunk driving is a misleading stereotype of the sort that should not be allowed to drive the engine of public policy. Public confidence in medical practice in general and organ transplantation in particular depends on the scientific validity and moral integrity of the policies adopted. Sound policies based on fact and sound ethical principles will prove publicly defensible. Shaping present health care policy on the basis of distorted public perceptions or prejudices will, in the long run, do more harm than good both to the nation at large and to the health care system.

Equal access for the medically suitable

The position that carefully selected, medically suitable alcoholic ESLD patients should be allowed to compete equally with medically suitable non-alcoholics has been developed by Cohen, Benjamin and the Ethics and Social Impact Committee of the Transplant and Health Policy Center (1991). As with the personal responsibility position, we first outline the argument and then critically assess it.

The argument

Alcohol-related ESLD is only one of a large number of illnesses that are, in some sense, attributable to personal conduct and, as a rule, treated without hesitation. Drivers in automobile accidents who are discovered to have been intoxicated or not wearing their seatbelts are given medical treatment regardless of whether either of these is causally responsible for their injuries. Heavy smokers suffering from lung cancer are also treated without question. Consider, too, coronary bypass candidates and heart transplantation candidates who disregarded their physicians' advice about tobacco, medication, diet and exercise; very sick diabetics who have not taken their insulin with sufficient regularity; AIDS patients who were intravenous drug abusers; and hypertensive patients who, despite repeated warnings, have refused to take antihypertensive medication and who have, as a result, developed end-stage renal failure.

We cannot single out alcoholics with ESLD as ineligible for certain forms of treatment because they may, in some sense, be personally responsible for their illness without doing the same for these other patients. The labored efforts of Moss and Siegler to distinguish alcoholic ESLD patients from these others do not, as indicated earlier, stand up to scrutiny. Alcoholic ESLD patients can justly be denied access to liver transplantation only as part of a comprehensive, systematic effort to withhold medical treatment from all patients shown to be personally responsible for their illnesses.

There are, moreover, significant obstacles to such an undertaking. Restricting treatment on the grounds of patients' personal responsibility for their illness would be extremely difficult to implement. It would, in the first place, involve highly intrusive investigations into patients' private lives. Second, it would often presume more than we can honestly claim to know about the degree of voluntariness underlying a patient's behavior. Can we, for example, be certain that all patients have the same will-power with regard to medically prudent behavior? At least two considerations should make us pause: (1) we have no direct access to, or way of measuring, another's will-power, and (2) most of us will, in reflecting on our own lives, acknowledge that our will-power has varied from time to time and from context to context. We should, as a result, exhibit some humility in judging the voluntariness of others, especially if such judgments are to be the basis of withholding needed, lifesaving medical treatment.

Justice requires that similar illnesses be treated similarly unless there is clear and conclusive evidence of relevant differences in terms of patient responsibility and the criteria employed in making these discriminations are uniformly and comprehensively applied. The burden of proof is thus on those who would argue that alcoholic patients, sick enough to need a new liver and who, after careful medical, psychiatric and social evaluation, are judged likely to benefit from this limited resource, should not be assessed on the same basis as other patients. This is, for reasons given above, a difficult burden to discharge.

Assessment of the argument

Although this position seems to us more plausible than the personal responsibility position, it may be criticized by some as still too restrictive and by others as too lenient. Consider, first, an argument to the effect that in subjecting alcoholics to a special evaluation with respect to their continued drinking, the equal access position may be discriminating against the least fortunate or poorest groups of alcoholics. In the USA, Makela and Room report:

> The balance of the system is tipping away from publicly funded institutions and towards private hospitals, often run for profit by corporate chains. These private institutions serve only those who can pay their expensive fees through health insurance or corporate or family wealth, and thus automatically exclude the poor or unemployed heavy drinker. In the publicly funded treatment centers, there has been a rapid transformation in function and clientele. Under pressure of budget cuts, many treatment agencies are rapidly becoming correctional centers, financed by their clients rather than the state as adjuncts to the criminal court system, (Makela and Room, 1985, p. 3).

The problem, they add, is aggravated by an ethically questionable 'de facto policy of encouraging alcohol consumption and organizing our social life around it, while stringently penalizing the individual drinker . . . ' (Makela and Room, 1985, p. 4). How, under such circumstances, can we justify not only giving a lower priority for receiving a new liver to alcoholic ESLD patients but also requiring them to undergo a special evaluation to determine future abstinence? 'A drunkard,' Makela and Room conclude, 'should have the same entitlements and rights as any other citizen similarly situated' (Makela and Room, 1985, p. 4).

There is something to be said for this objection. It should, at very least, temper self-righteous censure of all patients with alcohol-related ESLD. It does not follow, however, that we violate the rights of such patients by assessing the likelihood that they will be able to comply with the follow-up care required of transplant recipients. Transplantable organs are, in the words of a National Task Force, 'a national resource to be used for the public good' (Task Force on Organ Transplantation, 1986, p. 86). Thus the transplantation system has obligations not only to potential recipients but also to the society at large and to those individuals and families that have donated transplantable livers, to allocate these limited, lifesaving resources fairly and efficiently (Ethics Committee United Network for Organ Sharing (UNOS), 1992). An efficient allocation is one that contributes to aggregate patient survival. Among the relevant considerations in determining the likelihood of success in liver transplantation in alcohol-related ESLD patients is whether we have good reason to believe that they will be able to stop drinking. This requirement is more a medical than moralistic consideration. That it does not unjustly discriminate against alcoholics becomes clear when we envisage the possibility of two alcohol-related ESLD patients competing for the same transplantable liver. Suppose careful investigation has determined that one patient is much less likely to resume heavy drinking than the other. Would we not, other things being equal, be more justified in allocating the liver to the patient more likely to comply with the demands of follow-up care than the one less likely to do so?

The remaining objections to the equal access position come from a different direction: from those who maintain that it is too accepting of alcohol-related ESLD patients. The first objection expresses concern with the possible effects of public perception if carefully selected alcoholic patients were allowed to compete equally with non-alcoholics. Even if there were no plausible justification for the personal responsibility position's nearly categorical preference for non-alcoholic over carefully selected alcoholic liver transplant candidates, the possibility remains that the public's opposition to equal treatment might lead to a precipitous decline in overall support for liver transplantation. That the policy is right in principle would then be hollow consolation to potential recipients who, as a matter of fact, would be denied access to liver transplantation because of the significant erosion in public support.

The second objection centers on possible cases in which it seems intuitively wrong to allow someone whose ESLD is almost certainly attributable to his or her heavy drinking to complete equally with someone whose liver failure we are equally certain is wholly outside his or her control. 'It is fairer to give a child dying of biliary atresia an opportunity for a first normal liver', Moss and Siegler argue, 'than it is to give a patient with ARESLD [alcohol-related ESLD] who was born with a normal liver a second one' (Moss and Siegler, 1991, p. 1297). By itself, the intuitive appeal of this claim is quite powerful. Yet we must be careful about basing public policy on generalizations from particular cases because they are not always representative. With this case, for example, it is hard to determine how much of one's visceral agreement is attributable to the child's age and how much to the fact that the second patient is an alcoholic. Other things being equal, there are reasons of justice, as well as utility, for giving some priority to younger over older patients. Of two equally qualified candidates for a liver, the younger has had less opportunity to live than the older and therefore may have a greater claim to the organ based on considerations of justice. If the younger candidate is also likely to live longer with the new liver than the older candidate, a greater claim may also be justified on utilitarian grounds. One ought, then, to ask oneself if the example would have as much intuitive force if both patients were the same age. Moreover, generalizations from unrepresentative cases may lead to distorted public policy. If the two candidates were Mother Teresa and Charles Manson, one might be tempted to opt for criteria of social worth rather than some combination of medical utility, medical urgency and first-come, first-served. Other pairs of examples would not be nearly so clear and, as a result, provide considerable embarrassment for such a generalization. Still, there may be something troubling about giving no consideration whatever to the fact that of two competing equally qualified liver recipients one could have done absolutely nothing to have averted his or her ESLD whereas the other, an alcoholic, may have done something to have prevented his or her ESLD. This leads to a possible compromise position.

A compromise

Is there a possible middle ground between the personal responsibility and equal access positions? While acknowledging a sense in which many, if not most, alcoholic patients are responsible for their ESLD in a way in which non-alcoholic patients are not, a compromise position places less weight on this factor in determining access to transplantation than does the personal responsibility position.

The argument

There is something to be said for the claim that alcoholic patients generally bear some responsibility for their ESLD that non-alcoholic patients generally do not. Yet this observation must be tempered by a number of other factors. It is, for example, difficult in individual cases to determine whether a particular alcoholic patient had the will-power or actual opportunity to seek effective treatment for alcoholism. Moreover, it seems arbitrary to single out alcoholic ESLD as a condition for having a significantly lower priority to needed medical treatment without doing the same for other severe illnesses – such as, for example, those precipitated by a failure to take prescribed medication – for which individuals bear a comparable level of personal responsibility. Finally, assigning absolute priority to non-alcoholic over alcoholic ESLD patients with respect to access to transplantation ignores other important values and considerations in organ allocation.

The personal responsibility position, one might say, places too much weight on a patient's alcoholism in determining access to transplantation, whereas the equal access position gives it too little weight. What is needed is a compromise, a position that gives some consideration to alcohol consumption as a likely cause of a patient's ESLD but that does not make it an absolute or decisive consideration.

Priority for non-alcoholic ESLD patients can be either absolute or a matter of degree. Advocates of the personal responsibility position recommend that priority be absolute. Alcoholic ESLD patients are either in or out. If they were not previously been offered therapy for their alcoholism or if there were no suitable non-alcoholic recipients they are in. Otherwise they are out. This is simplistic in the light of the many different values involved in organ allocation and the actual process for allocating livers outlined above. Rather than allowing alcoholism to override all other considerations in liver allocation, it ought to included as one, but only one, element in the overall process. How can this be accomplished?

The fact that a patient's ESLD is likely to have been caused by heavy drinking might be factored into the allocation system directly or indirectly. The system might, for example, indirectly prioritize some non-alcoholics over alcoholics by assigning a certain number of allocation points in inverse proportion to age. This would give some advantage, but not absolute advantage, to younger (presumably non-alcoholic) over older candidates. Other things being equal, a child suffering from biliary atresia would, on this basis, receive a new liver before an abstinent, carefully selected alcoholic patient. More directly, the system could award a certain number of points (2? 3? 4?) to non-alcoholic patients for clearly having had no control over succumbing to liver failure. This sort of tilt would give a modest edge to non-alcoholic candidates but it would be a matter of degree, not absolute. It would not be decisive. For example, an alcoholic ESLD patient who receives significantly more points on grounds of blood type, time on the waiting list and degree of medical urgency might still receive a new liver before a particular non-alcoholic patient.

Thus this third position more or less splits the difference between the other two. It acknowledges that there is some sense in which alcoholic ESLD patients are likely to be responsible for their illness in a way that non-alcoholic patients are not. Yet at the same time, it tempers its judgment by making this only one factor in determining access to transplantation. In so doing it not only acknowledges the uncertainty of attributions of personal responsibility but it is also more responsive to the complex, multivalued nature of liver allocation than the personal responsibility position.

Assessment of the argument

This position is still likely to do an injustice to some alcoholic patients who, on examination, can be shown to bear no personal responsibility whatsoever for their ESLD. Consider, again, someone born into abusive and hopeless circumstances, who began drinking heavily at the age of 12 and was not able to bring his or her alcohol consumption under control until some years later, by which time ESLD had developed. Can we hold the perhaps quite understandable, self-destructive behavior of such adolescents against them at a later stage in life when, with the aid of greater maturity, social support and more hopeful circumstances, they are able to pull their lives together and stop their drinking? Though an improvement over the personal responsibility position in this regard, the compromise will still be making punitive judgments in a situation where none should be made.

In addition, unless included as part of a more comprehensive, general effort to incorporate personal responsibility for illness as a criterion for access to care, the compromise position arbitrarily and discriminatorily singles out alcoholics for special negative treatment, attenuated though it may be. If the issue is actually personal responsibility, and not alcoholism, the proposal should be part of a larger, more general heath care policy.

Finally, the system already tilts against carefully selected alcoholic liver transplant candidates. There is no need for further penalties, even the more modest ones proposed by the proposed compromise. The additional medical, psychiatric and social workups required to determine whether such patients, are in fact, good risks for transplantation puts them at a comparative disadvantage with other patients whose ESLD and need for a liver transplant may have been diagnosed at the same time. Thus any additional factors, such as adding a couple of UNOS points to the totals of non-alcoholic patients compounds an existing handicap borne by alcoholic patients. There is no need for an additional penalty because, given the very nature of the special selection process, alcoholics do not in fact compete equally with non-alcoholic patients for available livers.

Conclusion

The personal responsibility position is, as we have shown, irreparably flawed. It employs a double standard in singling out alcoholics from others whose illnesses are comparably self-induced, it presumes more knowledge about voluntariness than we can actually obtain, it is insensitive to the wide variety of cases in which alcohol consumption may be related to ESLD and it ignores the importance of other values in organ allocation. Both the equal access and compromise positions are more justifiable from an ethical point of view than the personal responsibility position. Choosing between them is, however, more difficult. While each is preferable to the personal responsibility position, neither is free of problems. Yet an inability to show that one of these positions is clearly more justifiable than the other may make little difference in practice. Even if one were to adopt the equal access position, the additional time required for adequate medical, psychiatric and social evaluation of the alcoholic patient may make the actual outcome practically indistinguishable from that of the compromise position.

References

Aaron, H. J. and Schwartz, W. B. (1984). *The Painful Prescription: Rationing Hospital Care.* Washington, DC: The Brookings Institution.

Beresford, T. P., Turcotte, J. G., Tsakis, A. G., Merion, R.M., Burtch, G., Blow, F.C., Campbell, D.A., Brower, K.J., Coffman, K. and Lucey, M.R. (1990). A rational approach to liver transplantation for the alcoholic patient. *Psychosomatics*, **31**, 241–54.

Cohen, C., Benjamin, M. and the Ethics and Social Impact Committee of the Transplant and Health Policy Center (1991). Alcoholics and liver transplantation. *Journal of the American Medical Association*, **265**, 1299–1301.

Ethics Committee, United Network for Organ Sharing (1992). General principles for allocating human organs and tissues. *Transplantation Proceedings*, **24**, 2227–35.

Lucey, M. R. and Beresford, T. P. (1992). Alcoholic liver disease: to transplant or not to transplant? *Alcohol and Alcoholism*, **27**, 103–8.

Lucey, M. R., Merion, R. M., Henley, K. S., Campbell, D.A., Turcotte, J.G., Nosttant, T.T., Blow, F.C. and Beresford, T.P. (1992). Selection for and outcome of liver transplantation in alcoholic liver disease. *Gastroenterology*, **102**, 1736–41.

Makela, K. and Room, R. (1985). Alcohol policy and the rights of the drunkard. *Alcoholism, Clinical and Experimental Research*, **9**, 2–5.

Morris, H. (1968). Persons and punishment. *The Monist*, **52**, 475–501.

Moss, A. H. and Siegler, M. (1991). Should alcoholics compete equally for liver transplantation? *Journal of the American Medical Association*, **265**, 1295–8.

Scharschmidt, B. F. (1984). Human liver transplantation: analysis of data on 54 patients from four centers. *Hepatology*, **4**:95S–101S.

Starzl, T. E., Van Thiel, D., Tsakis, A. G., Iwatsuki, S., Todo, S., March, J.W., Kowden, B., Staschak, S. and Stieber (1988). Orthotopic liver transplantation for alcoholic cirrhosis. *Journal of the American Medical Association*, **260**, 2542–4.

Task Force on Organ Transplantation (1986). *Organ Transplantation: Issues and Recommendations*. Washington, DC: US Department of Health and Human Services.

INDEX